Helmut Re

GENTLE EXERCISES
FOR
BETTER HEALTH

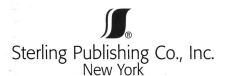

Sterling Publishing Co., Inc.
New York

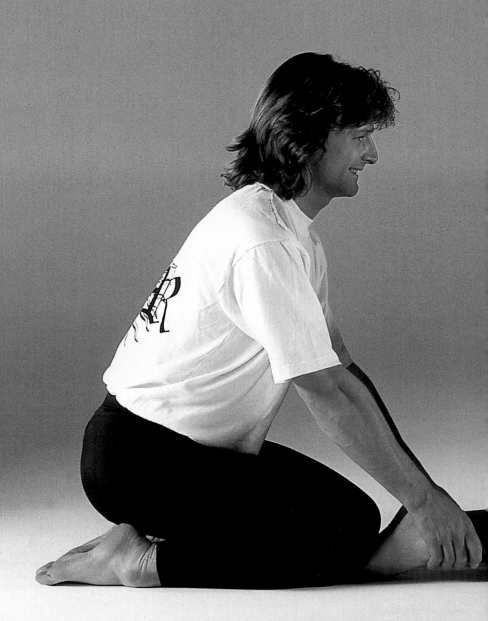

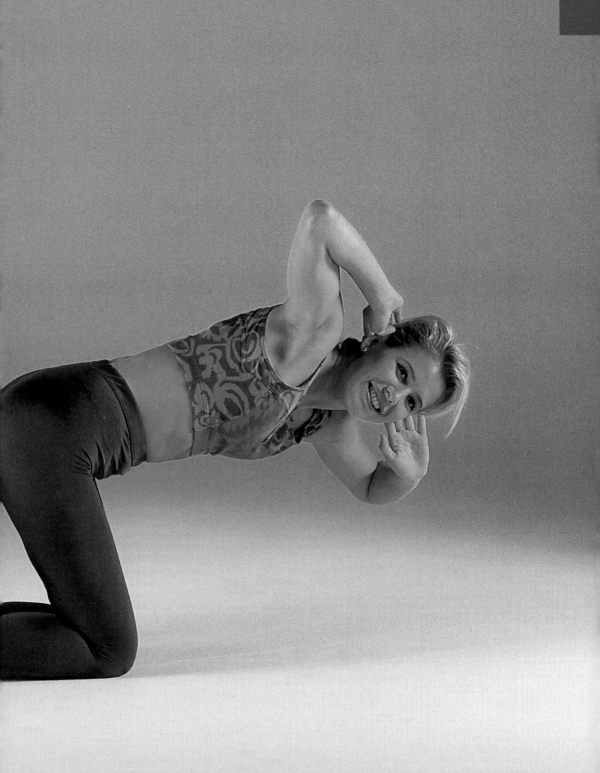

Exercises demonstrated by Fiona Bendelack and Michael Mayer
Photographs: Ulli Seer
Layout: Atelier Steinbicker, Munich
Production: Friedrich Wilhelm Bonhagen
Translated by Eva-Maria Sawers

Helmut Reichardt was born in Augsburg, Germany, in 1953. He studied at the Technical University in Darmstadt, where he received a teaching certificate for the high school level in 1977. After training as a physiotherapist, Reichardt resumed his studies at the University of Tübingen and at the same time trained as a sports physiotherapist. In 1985, he received his master's degree in sports education and biology. Until 1989, he was an assistant lecturer in the Department of Sports Science at the University of Tübingen. Since 1981, he has worked as a physiotherapist in competitive sports (for the Federal League for Volleyball and the national squad of the German Basketball Association). Since 1989, he has also worked as a freelance adviser on sports and health matters, and he is an endurance athlete himself.

Library of Congress Cataloging-in-Publication Data

10 9 8 7 6 5 4 3 2 1

Published by Sterling Publishing Company, Inc.
387 Park Avenue South, New York, N.Y. 10016
Originally published in Germany under the title *Schongymnastik: das Übungsprogramm für Beweglichkeit, Leistungsfähigkeit und Wohlbefinden* and © 1996 by BLV Verlagsgesellschaft mbH
English translation © 1999 by Sterling Publishing Co., Inc.
Distributed in Canada by Sterling Publishing
c/o Canadian Manda Group, One Atlantic Avenue, Suite 105
Toronto, Ontario, Canada M6K 3E7
Distributed in Great Britain and Europe by Cassell PLC
Wellington House, 125 Strand, London WC2R 0BB, England
Distributed in Australia by Capricorn Link (Australia) Pty Ltd.
P.O. Box 6651, Baulkham Hills, Business Centre, NSW 2153, Australia
Manufactured in the United States of America
All rights reserved

Sterling ISBN 0-8069-9451-7

Contents

Preface

Gymnastic exercises have been used for thousands of years. In more recent times, this form of physical activity has been influenced by various fashionable programs, such as aerobics, stretching, body-shaping, and calisthenics, all of which originated in America.

Through his publications, Helmut Reichardt has initiated a new line of development over the last couple of decades that is independent of fashionable trends and focuses on the health and well-being of the individual. These "gentle exercises" are a successful synthesis of applied anatomical and physiological knowledge.

The easy, therapeutic exercises in this book, inspired by those used in physiotherapy, have a bearing on metabolic, preventive, stabilizing, and rehabilitative processes, and thus have great importance for our health.

They gently work on all the muscles, tendons, and joints; they maintain and improve mobility and, in some cases, strength; they alleviate everyday aches and pains and rectify muscular imbalances; and they provide preparation for, and a supplement to, almost any sports activity.

Although these exercises are no substitute for a course of physiotherapy prescribed by your doctor, they do offer an easy way to become fit and healthy and to stay that way. With his gentle exercises, sports physiotherapist Helmut Reichardt has created a program reflecting a functional view of posture and movement. Doing these exercises will give you a sense of physical and mental well-being, and allow you to rediscover your body more and more as you train.

This book has proved a great success in Germany, where it is now in its eighth edition, and is highly recommended to all athletes, gymnasts, sports teachers, physiotherapists, and indeed all those who care about their health.

Dr. Manfred Grosser,
Chair of Mobility and Training Science,
Technical University of Munich

Introduction

There is certainly nothing new in taking a functional view of the locomotor system (the totality of muscles, tendons, and joints) and asking how different joints and muscles work. The study of traditional functional anatomy and the realization of its findings in therapeutic exercises have been providing evidence of this for years.

In the realm of sports, however, the human body is seen more in the context of its ability to perform complex movements. An approach that examines individual joint and muscle movements is not very common. In gymnastics, such ideas have indeed been put forward from time to time over the years, but they have been applied to its own sphere rather than in influencing training procedures in other sports.

Only in recent years has there been increasing interest among athletes in gymnastic exercises that aim to exploit specific functions of the locomotor system. "Stretching" as a new type of exercise is just one example of this. In addition, terms such as "functional exercises" have been coined, and have gained increasing importance in the sports world.

In this process, many traditional exercises have been examined critically and their effects questioned. As a result, some people in the sports field became uncertain of the value of particular exercises and soon began to seek alternatives.

The functional method, upon which the exercises in this book are based, is an alternative attracting more and more practitioners. The functional method is described more fully below, and, by means of exercise examples, individual elements of an exercise are viewed using this approach. These points are referred to in the main part of the book in the commentary on the exercises.

The introduced exercises always make use of the basic movements of the different parts of the body. In this way, it is possible to improve the strength and mobility of specific muscles despite the workouts being kept deliberately simple. The different variants of the exercises make it possible for both those who are not in training and those who participate actively in sports to find the right level.

The range of exercises presented here will increase your energy as well as your overall feeling of well-being, alleviating common aches and pains and countering the overuse of certain muscles in competitive sports.

Even in such cases where the individual muscle groups are made to work very hard, the locomotor system and especially the spine are not subjected to any strain if the exercise is done correctly—hence, the choice of the term "gentle exercises."

The Functional Approach

If an exercise regime is regarded functionally—that is, from the point of view of the functions it is to perform—then those exercises that aim to increase the strength and mobility of the muscles are the most important. In order to establish what effect an exercise has, we have to look at both the content of the exercise, meaning the movements themselves, and the way the exercise is executed. In this context, it can be helpful to have knowledge of how our bodies work, and particularly our muscles.

Analyzing Exercises Functionally

The Jackknife

A popular toning, or strengthening, exercise for the abdominal muscles is the "jackknife" (Fig. 1). If you observe the sequence of movements, it is clear that what is involved above all is a bending at the hips, and so it is the flexors of the hips that are used primarily in this exercise.

The abdominal muscles here have the important task of drawing the upper torso toward the pelvis. However, if the muscles are not strong enough to do this satisfactorily, then in order to compensate an increased flexing of the pelvis and arching of the lower back will occur at the beginning of the exercise. The jackknife then becomes a mere hip-flexing exercise, which in cases of a weak initial effort from the abdominal muscles leads to an excessive load on the lumbar vertebrae.

If the abdominal muscles are to be used more efficiently then to suit the way they function, the main feature of the exercise has to be the flexing of the upper torso.

The way the hip-flexing muscles are used is restricted by the choice of a suitable starting position (Fig. 2).

The function of the abdominal muscles ceases here when the shoulders and the thoracic vertebrae have been lifted off the floor. However,

Fig. 1
For the jackknife exercise, a powerful effort is required from the hip-flexing muscles. Because of the anatomical process involved, sudden stress on these muscles frequently causes an arching of the back.

Fig. 2
Tensing the hip flexors is a suitable starting position for executing the movements. This enables the abdominal muscle to be used in the appropriate way.

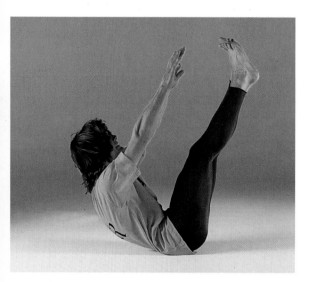

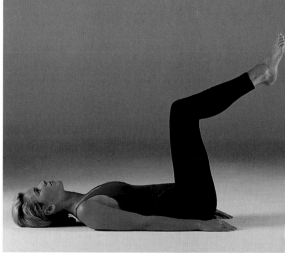

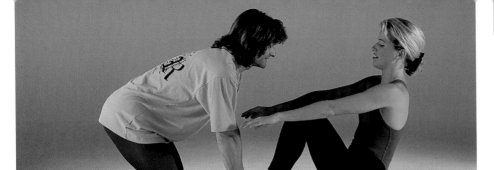

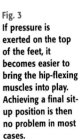

Fig. 3
If pressure is exerted on the top of the feet, it becomes easier to bring the hip-flexing muscles into play. Achieving a final sit-up position is then no problem in most cases.

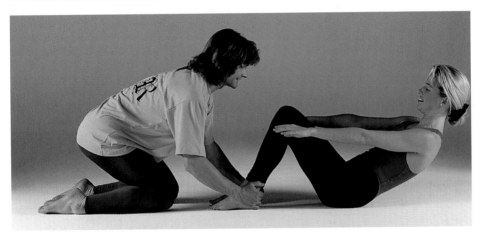

Fig. 4
If there is no assistance for the hip muscles, a sit-up can no longer be achieved, or only be achieved with difficulty.

this requires a strong initial effort, which is often not possible (see page 15).

You can return to the sitting position only by using the hip flexors, although this rarely works.

Energetic execution of the jackknife exercise has another drawback: The muscles involved at the beginning of the movement are subjected to powerful exertion, which leads to an accelerated movement of the legs and the torso. The final position is then usually achieved without much further effort, which is not the aim of the exercise.

In contrast, when the exercise is performed very slowly, the muscles involved are more evenly stressed, producing better, more gentle effects.

Sit-ups

Another popular exercise for toning the abdominal muscles is the sit-up. If, at the start, both legs are bent and held down by a partner using pressure on the top of the feet, it is usually possible to regain the sitting position (Fig. 3). However, if the partner holds the ankles instead, the sitting position is very difficult to achieve. The exercise is complete when the shoulder blades are raised and the thoracic vertebrae curved (Fig. 4), which means the abdominal muscles are being used correctly.

In the first version of the exercise (Fig. 3), the pressure applied to the top of the feet affects the whole relevant muscle chain, activating the hip-flexing and the abdominal muscles. The bending movement is a combined flexing of the hips and the upper torso.

In the second version (Fig. 4), the hip flexors are not activated due to pressure in a different place, and it is primarily the abdominal muscles that come into play. However, after the torso has been flexed, the motor function of the abdominal muscles ceases and it is no longer possible to sit up. The effect of the restraining pressure on the muscles can be demonstrated even more impressively with the following example.

While lying on your back with your legs extended, press your toes into your partner's hands, which support them. If the relevant muscles are tensed sufficiently, then no effort is required from your partner when lifting your body off the floor as if it were a plank of wood (Fig. 5), because as

before a whole chain of muscles is activated.

Therefore, it is clear that it's not only the choice of the starting and final positions that is important. Depending on the way the starting position is steadied by a partner or some other aid, the groups of muscles involved in the execution of the movement also change. In addition, the effects the particular exercise has depend just as much on the way it is carried out, and especially on the speed of the movement.

Stretching Muscles the Right Way

An example from a range of stretching exercises will demonstrate that here, too, it can be useful to think in terms of function.

Stretching the front of the thigh is usually performed by standing upright and pulling the foot toward the buttock with the hand on that side. Complete stretching of the relevant group of

Fig. 5
As you press your toes into your partner's hands, which are holding them, the whole chain of muscles along the back of your legs and your torso is activated.

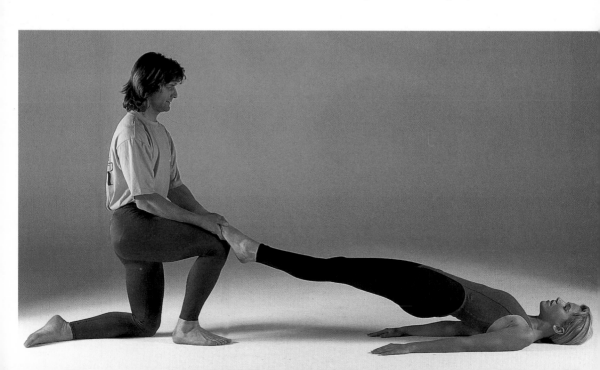

muscles will not be achieved if the final position is that shown in Fig. 6, as is frequently the case in practice.

One part of the quadriceps muscle on the front of the thigh extends over the hip joint, and its function is to flex. This part can be stretched with the hip joint fully extended only if the knee joint is bent at the same time.

In Fig. 6, a compensatory movement can clearly be seen—that is, a flexing at the hip.

A more functionally appropriate method of stretching the front of the thigh is demonstrated in Fig. 7.

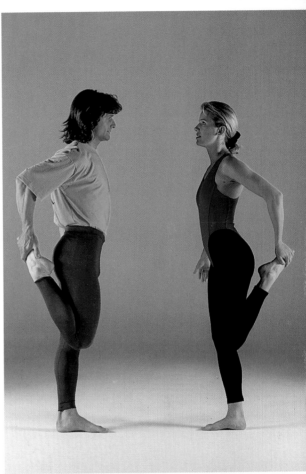

Fig. 6
Stretching the straight thigh muscle is not correct functionally if the pelvis is inclined in the final position.

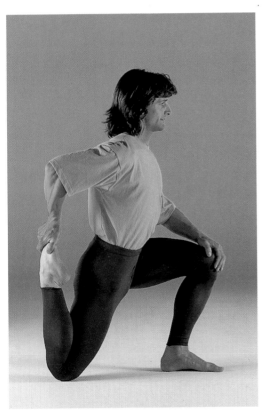

Fig. 7
Functional stretching of the straight thigh muscle without any compensatory movement.

Correcting Muscular Imbalance

As mentioned previously, exercises based on function concentrate on those that strengthen the muscles and increase mobility. It's important not only to get the content and the execution of the individual exercises right, but also to combine these toning and stretching exercises correctly.

At this point, we need to take into consideration the "muscular imbalances" that can occur in a muscle system. If in one part of the body, due to either lack of activity or excessive strain on one muscle, an imbalance occurs between the strength of one muscle group and the ability of another to stretch, this can lead to functional disorders.

Muscular imbalance can be illustrated by the following example: Apart from their motor function when flexing the upper torso, the abdominal muscles also have the task of holding the pelvis upright. If the abdominal muscles no longer have sufficient tension, the pelvis is inclined forward. This causes the lumbar vertebrae to change position, resulting in what is often referred to as a "hollow back."

This faulty posture is accompanied in most cases by a shortening, and thus poor, stretching ability of the hip-flexing muscles. Due to its location in the body, this group of muscles can aggravate the inclination of the pelvis and therefore also the hollow back.

Toning the abdominal muscles by itself would do little to rectify this imbalance; it is always necessary to stretch the hip-flexing muscles at the same time.

Executing Toning Exercises

We can make some general assumptions regarding the execution of toning exercises using the functional approach. The following recommendations can be made for those toning exercises aimed primarily at the sets of muscles liable to become weak:

▶ Always exercise slowly and correctly.

▶ Never try to speed through or bypass the movement specified.

▶ Move on to more advanced exercises only when you have mastered the simple ones.

Some types of exercise involve holding a position (static exercises). The following principles apply to them:

▶ The muscle-tensing position should be held for 5 to 6 seconds.

▶ After the initial two to three repetitions, work up to a maximum of six repetitions.

▶ While holding the position, breathe calmly and evenly, but if this is impossible, hold the position for the length of only one exhalation.

For those exercises that involve movement (dynamic exercises), the following principles apply:

▶ The movement is repeated slowly five to six times without a break (from the start to the point where you come out of the final position should take about 2 seconds).

▶ Start with a single series of exercises, working up to three over time.

▶ If you can perform the five to six repetitions without effort, then add a pause of 2 to 3 seconds before going back to the starting position.

▶ Using this method of exercising, the workout should be increased to three series of exercises, each with five to six repetitions.

Your target is to achieve the following:

▶ Get from the starting position to the final position in about 2 seconds, hold it for 2 seconds, and then return to the starting position in about 2 seconds.

▶ The whole exercise routine need not take longer than 15 to 20 minutes.

▶ Do the exercises as frequently as possible (at least twice a week).

Executing Stretching Exercises

Recommendations can also be made regarding stretching exercises. As with the toning exercises, this advice will be supplemented in the exercise descriptions in the main body of the book. We are concerned here with stretching exercises for muscle groups liable to shortening.

It's important to take the following into consideration:

▶ Stretching the muscles should be carried out in a slow and measured fashion.

▶ The appropriate final position should be held for 10 to 15 seconds.

▶ To achieve good results, repeat each exercise two to three times.

▶ Stretching must not cause pain.

▶ The held form of muscular stretching is the initial, preparatory stretching performed before any sports activity.

When you begin the exercises, you will find instructions to follow, in addition to these general principles. Experience has indicated that certain exercises are often done incorrectly, and, for them, there is an illustration showing the common mistake with relevant comments. For all the exercises that don't work the muscle system symmetrically—that is, they can be performed on either the right or the left side—instructions are given for one side only.

In selecting functional toning and stretching exercises for your own routine, adjustments should be made according to your personal strengths and weaknesses. For this reason, you will find exercise tests to help you determine your level. (A couple of examples of exercise tests are included in the section that follows.)

At the end of the book, there are at-a-glance exercise routines for both beginners and those with more experience that summarize the main areas for the use of function-based exercises and provide useful combinations of stretching and toning exercises.

Practical Application: Exercise Tests

Exercise tests are included in the book to help you select the best routines for yourself. It has to be stressed that none of these tests can pinpoint existing deficiencies with absolute certainty. They are only a means of suggesting appropriate exercises. Furthermore, they can be used as a check on your progress.

If in the strength test the final position is reached without effort, then you can go on to more difficult exercises. This will be specified in each case in the text. But if weaknesses become evident, then the simpler versions should be chosen.

Stretching exercises are not graded as to difficulty, because the intensity is determined by the individual's subjective judgment. The selection of the exercises is governed by individual capabilities. If deficiencies are discovered when testing the ability to

stretch, then the appropriate stretching positions should be used.

Testing the Hip-Flexing and Abdominal Muscles

Let us clarify this point further by using the example of the hip-flexing and abdominal muscles already mentioned. To test the stretching ability of the hip flexors, lie on the floor and pull one leg as close to your ribs as you can. The other leg remains stretched out, and gravity keeps it in line with the extended hip (Fig. 8).

If the pulling on the bent leg lifts the extended leg off the floor, this may well be caused by a lack of stretching ability in the hip-flexing muscles on the side of this extended leg. You should therefore choose exercises from pages 73 to 77 that will stretch the relevant muscles.

The test may also be influenced by an amply proportioned torso or by well-developed leg muscles. It is therefore only to be taken as a rough guide.

Fig. 8
Testing the stretching ability of the hip-flexing muscles:
Lying on your back, clasp one leg with both hands and pull it toward your torso as far as you can. If the extended leg lifts off the floor, the most likely explanation is shortened hip-flexing muscles on that side.

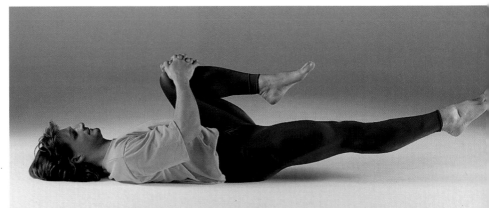

To test the strength of the abdominal muscles, slowly raise the upper torso with the legs bent at the knees. Your hands meanwhile slide along the floor toward your heels. If you can manage to lift your head, shoulders, and thoracic vertebrae, then the abdominal muscles are strong enough. If you can do the same movement with your hands at the base of your neck (Fig. 9), then your abdominal muscles can be assumed to be quite strong. It is important that this test is carried out very slowly and accurately.

If you can only lift your head and shoulders off the floor, your abdominal muscles are probably weak (Fig. 10). The relevant toning exercises for the abdominal muscles start on page 16.

In the next section, various exercises are described for improving the stability of the muscle system, and are aimed in particular at muscle groups that tend to weaken (see page 12). All the exercises are kept simple so that they can be done any time at home without complicated equipment.

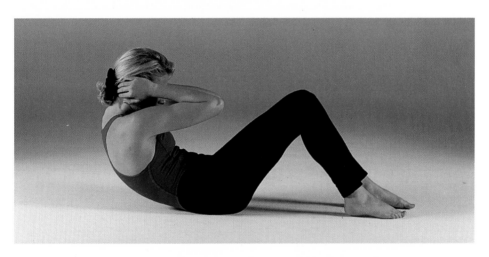

Fig. 9
Testing the strength of the abdominal muscles: Lying on your back with your legs bent at the knees, raise your upper torso slowly with your hands at the base of your neck. If you can lift your head, shoulders, and thoracic vertebrae off the floor, your abdominal muscles are very strong.

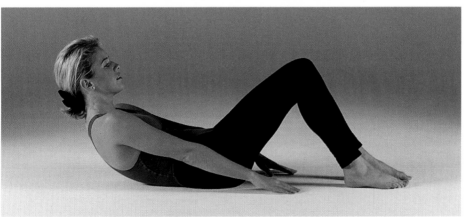

Fig. 10
When the abdominal muscles are lacking in strength, it is only possible to reach this final position.

Exercises for Improving the Body's Equilibrium

Strengthening the Abdominal Muscles

The condition of the abdominal muscles can be tested as described on the previous page. Strengthening is achieved with the second and subsequent exercises.

Exercise

To get a better idea of how the abdominal muscles affect the position of the pelvis and the spine, start with this simple exercise. Begin by lying on your back with your legs bent at the hips and the knees. Your arms lie bent at right angles behind your head.

Fig. 11
Lying on your back with your legs bent, place your arms behind your head with your elbows bent at right angles.

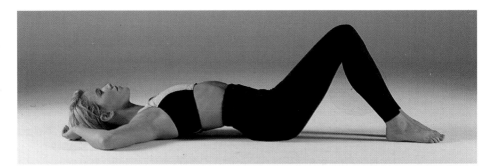

Fig. 12
Press the lumbar vertebrae against the floor with the aid of your abdominal muscles, and hold the position.

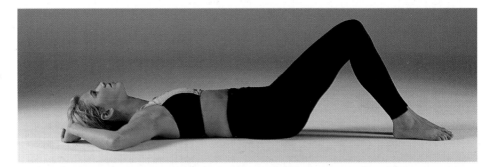

Fig. 13
Bend your legs, and slowly lift them as far as possible. Then return to the starting position, keeping your abdominal muscles tense.

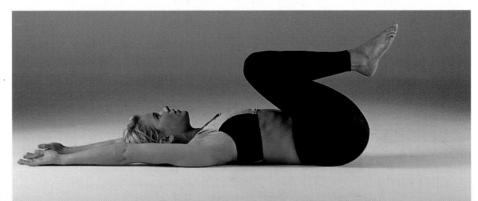

If you now press the lumbar spine against the floor, you can feel the tension in the abdominal muscles.

Without releasing the pressure exerted by the lumbar vertebrae on the floor, bend both legs and bring them up until the thighs touch the torso.

Then return your legs to the starting position, keeping the lumbar spine flattened against the floor until the movement is complete.

Repeat this simple exercise a few times, taking care to do it very slowly.

The guidelines given on page 12 apply to all the other body equilibrium exercises.

In all the following toning exercises for the muscles of the abdomen and the upper torso, the starting positions specified ensure that there is no strain on the lumbar spine.

At the beginning of the routine, always increase the pressure of the lumbar spine against the floor using your abdominal muscles before proceeding further with the exercises. This also applies to the exercises on this page.

Exercise
Lying on your back, bend both legs at the knees and lay your hands alongside your buttocks. Lift your head, and then slowly curve your spine, your hands being pulled slightly above the floor in the direction of your heels.

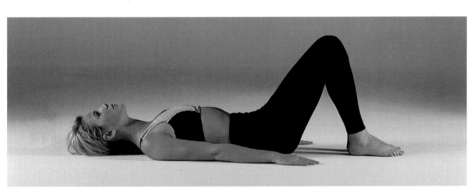

Fig. 14
Lying on your back with your legs bent, lay your hands flat alongside your buttocks.

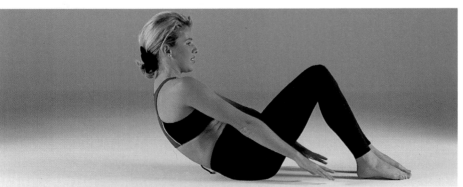

Fig. 15
Lift your head, and then slowly curve your spine

Advanced Version

In the more difficult form of the exercise, you hold your calves parallel to the floor and place your hands behind your head. You curve your spine as before, without your hands pulling on your head.

The position of your legs must not be changed.

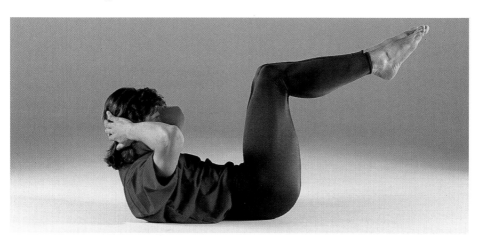

Fig. 16
Lying on your back, hold your calves parallel to the floor. Place your hands behind your head, and curve your spine as before.

Variation

This and the previous exercise can be varied by executing the movement diagonally. Move one shoulder at a time in the direction of the opposite hip.

This is a reminder that all exercises that can be executed to either the right or the left will only be described for one side.

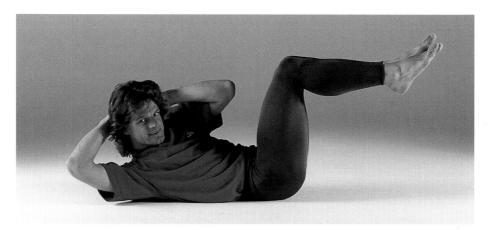

Fig. 17
A variation of the exercise: Move one shoulder in the direction of the opposite hip.

No-Load Position

If you find it difficult to control the position of the lumbar vertebrae, then the starting position can be made easier with the aid of a chair.

This "stepped positioning" is especially recommended if you have problems with your lower back.

Do the exercises as before, laying your hands alongside the buttocks in the easier version.

In the more difficult version, place your hands behind the head. Again, both versions can be varied by twisting the upper torso.

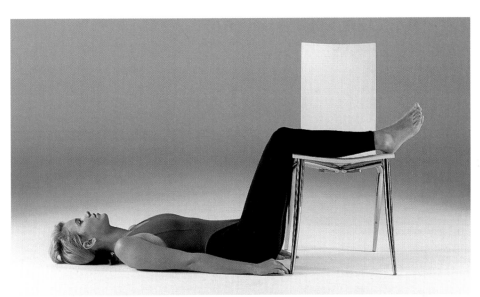

Fig. 18
Lying on your back, rest your calves on a chair. Depending on which variation is used, place your hands either alongside your buttocks or behind your head.

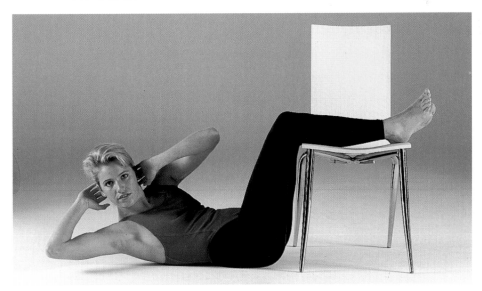

Fig. 19
The variation of the exercise is performed as before by moving one shoulder in the direction of the opposite hip.

Advanced Version

If the pelvis and the lumbar vertebrae are stabilized, then you can change the starting position as follows: Extend your legs, and hold them upward with the hip joint forming a right angle. Again, you must not change the position of the pelvis and the legs while executing any of the exercises described above from this position.

Be Careful!

Fig. 21 shows a popular exercise for toning the abdominal muscles, the scissors movement with extended legs off the floor. Here, a large part of the work is done by the hip-flexing muscles, as is the case with all exercises executed in a sitting position with straight legs.

Use the exercises in this section to execute a workout more specifically aimed at the abdominal muscles, especially when the strength test has revealed a weakness. Determining the strength of the abdominal muscles as described on page 14 can be supplemented with the following option.

Testing the Strength of the Abdominal Muscles

Test

Lying on your back, extend your legs and raise them to form a right angle at the hip joints. Place the backs of your hands under the lumbar vertebrae.

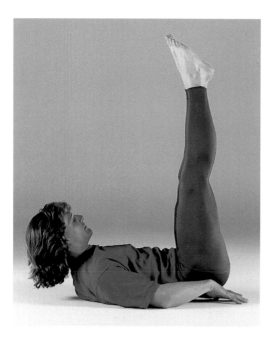

Fig. 20
This is another starting position, with your legs extended and held upward so that they form a right angle with the hip joints

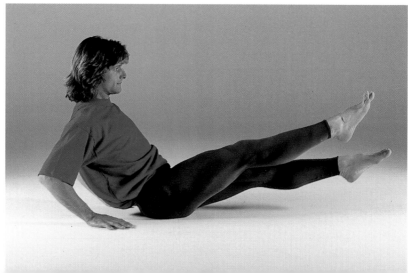

Fig. 21
All forms of exercise executed from a sitting position with legs extended put the hip-flexing muscles under a heavy strain.

Make your abdominal muscles work hard so that they are pressed against the backs of your hands (Fig. 22). Maintaining this contact, bring your legs (still extended) slowly down toward the floor (Fig. 23). If you can no longer keep the lumbar vertebrae flat (Fig. 24), then the test should be discontinued, bending your legs at the knees and bringing them back to the floor. If you can lower your extended legs a long way, this indicates that the abdominal muscles are stronger than if the start of the movement resulted in a hollow back. If you can lower your legs to the floor without any compensating movement of your pelvis, the stabilizing muscles are quite strong.

Note

Do not use this test as a regular exercise, because it puts considerable strain on the lumbar vertebrae.

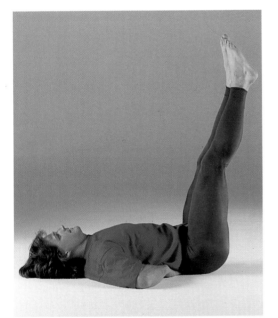

Fig. 22
Strength test for the abdominal muscles: Start by lying on your back, extending both legs to point vertically upward, and placing the backs of your hands under the lumbar vertebrae, with your head resting on the floor.

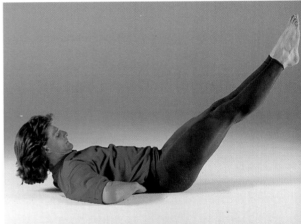

Fig. 23
Then, from the starting position, slowly lower your extended legs. Be sure that the strong pressure from the lumbar vertebrae against the backs of your hands maintains the contact with the hands as long as possible.

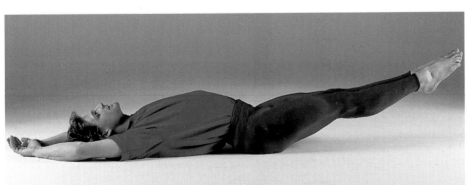

Fig. 24
If the lumbar vertebrae begin to lift off your hands, stop the test and return both legs to the floor. (To show the compensating movement clearly, the hands in the photo are in a different position.)

Strengthening the Abdominal Muscles by Lifting the Pelvis

In all the exercises shown so far, the abdominal muscles have been activated by curving the torso. If the torso is supported in the starting position and the legs and the pelvis are brought toward the torso, it is again the abdominal muscles that are made to work.

Exercise

Lying on your back, bend the hips and the knees so that your calves are held parallel to the floor. The pressure of your hands against the floor stabilizes the torso. Now lift the buttocks an inch or two off the floor so that your knees move upward. Raise your head, and fix your eyes on your knees.

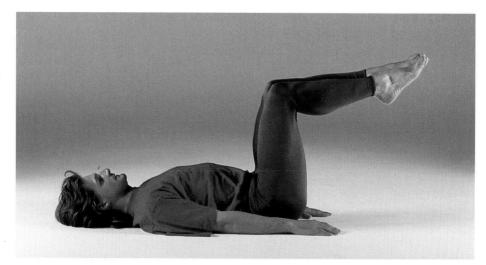

Fig. 25
Lying on your back, bend your hips and knees at right angles, and lay your hands alongside the buttocks.

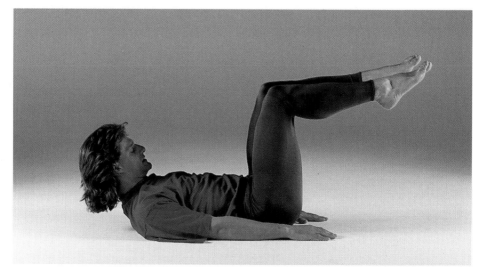

Fig. 26
Lift the buttocks slightly off the floor so that your knees move upward. Your eyes are directed at your thighs.

Important Note

You must not roll back onto your shoulders (as in the picture showing how not to do it), because the abdominal muscles are then no longer activated.

If you cannot manage to lift the buttocks out of the position shown in the photo, then you must flex your hip joints further to make this exercise easier. The more you stretch your legs, the more difficult this exercise will become.

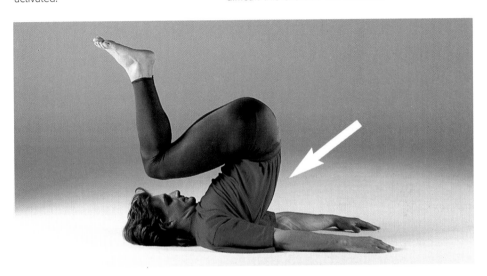

Fig. 27
How not to do it: The spine is curved too much so that the abdominal muscles are not made to work.

Variation

The form of the exercise shown in Fig. 26 can also be varied by moving the knees in the direction of the opposite shoulder.

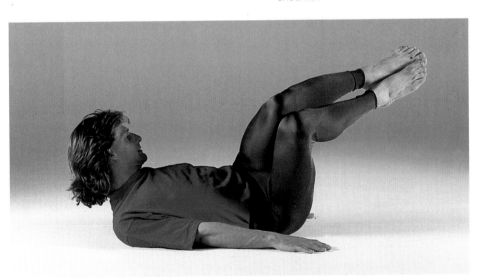

Fig. 28
In the raised position, you can rotate the pelvis alternately to the right and the left.

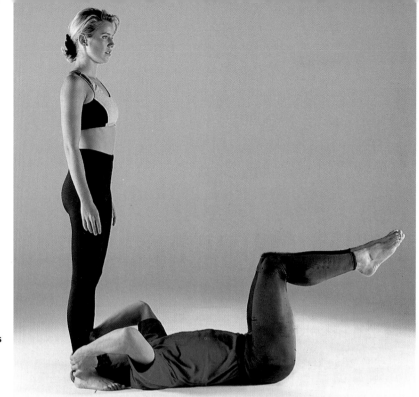

Fig. 29
**With both hands,
grasp the ankle joints
of your partner,
standing by your
head. The knee and
hip joints are flexed
at right angles.**

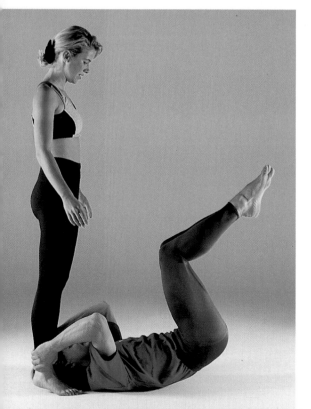

Fig. 30
**When your buttocks
lift off the floor, your
knees move upward.**

Working with a Partner

Because the upper arms are often not strong enough to stabilize the torso in the exercise on the previous page, it can also be done with the help of a partner.

With both hands, reach over your head to grasp the ankle joints of your partner for support.

The muscles are tensed as before by the slight lifting of the buttocks.

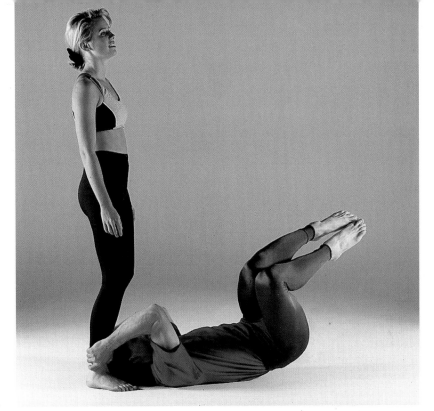

Fig. 31
In the raised
position, you can
rotate the pelvis
alternately to the
right and the left.

Fig. 32
In the raised
position, push one
knee at a time
higher than the
other.

Variations

The exercise can be varied by moving
the knees toward the opposite
shoulder. You can also raise one knee
higher than the other. By flexing your
hip joints more, the exercise can be
made easier, and by straightening
them, made more difficult. If no partner
is available, use a closet, door, or
similar object to provide support with
your hands above your head.

Another way specifically to make
your abdominal muscles work without
putting strain on the spine is by doing
the following exercise.

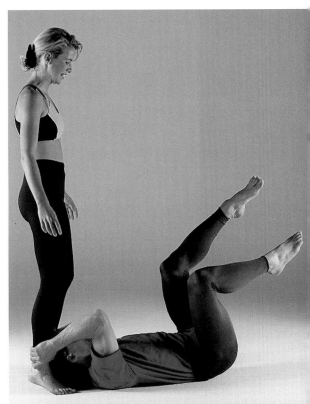

Exercise

Lying on your back, flex your hips and your knees until the palms of your hands touch your thighs. Place your hands slightly above the knees with the fingertips pointing toward each other. While pressing hard with your hands against your legs, resist this pressure with your legs.

Meanwhile, raise your head and fix your eyes on your knees.

Variation

This exercise can also be varied by reaching across with one hand to the diagonally opposite knee and increasing the tension by turning the upper torso slightly.

Because the degree of tension in the muscles is determined by their inherent resistance, it is not possible to prescribe any "dosage" for this exercise. And because the strain on the muscles of the upper torso can be great, remember to breathe freely.

Fig. 33
Lie on your back with your hips and knees bent, placing the palms of your hands on your thighs slightly above the knees.

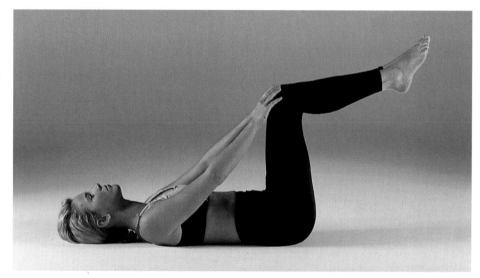

Fig. 34
While pressing hard with your hands against your thighs, resist this pressure with your thighs. Fix your eyes on your knees.

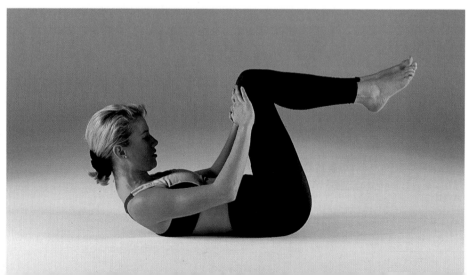

Toning Exercises with a Slight Prestretch for the Abdominal Muscles

All the abdominal muscle toning exercises described so far can also be performed with the aid of a roll of foam material or a tightly rolled-up mat. This should be put under the place where the thoracic and lumbar vertebrae meet, giving a slight prestretch to the abdominal muscles.

This starting position should be used only if it does not cause any pain.

If you suffer from a spinal defect, it can hurt. Otherwise, this position corresponds to the natural function of the spine.

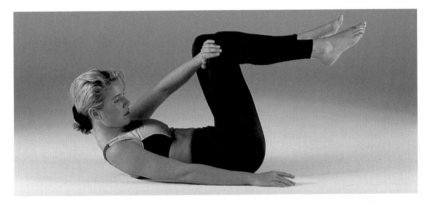

Fig. 35
Reach out one hand to meet the opposite knee, and press against it hard, while pushing with your knee in the opposite direction. Your head is raised.

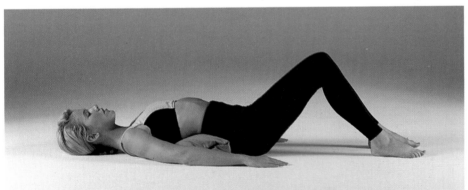

Fig. 36
Lie on your back, with your spine just above the pelvis supported from below with a roll. Bend your legs, and lay your hands alongside the buttocks.

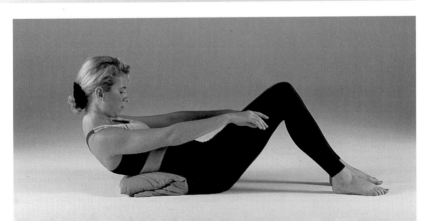

Fig. 37
From a supine position, slowly start to sit up, curving your spine. Your hands will be pushed in the direction of your feet.

Working with a Partner

If you find sitting up from a supine position with your legs bent impossible, a partner can stabilize the starting position by holding your heels.

Raising the pelvis with the hips and knees bent can also be achieved more easily with the help of a partner.

Fig. 38
Lie on your back, with your spine just above the pelvis supported from below with a roll, while your partner gives support at your heels. The curving of your spine is as before.

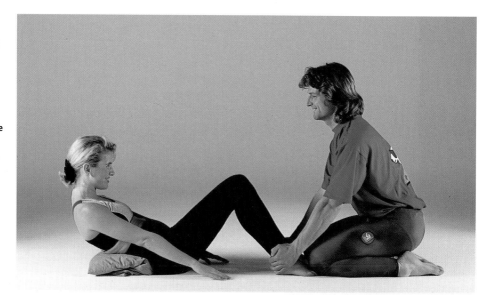

Fig. 39
In the more difficult form of the exercise, you place your hands behind your head.

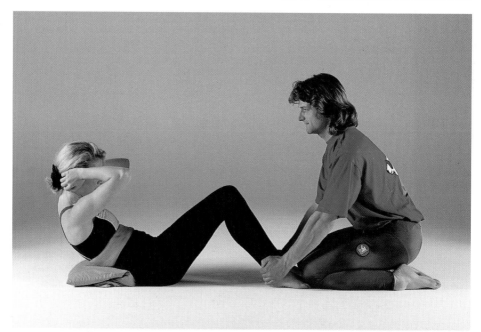

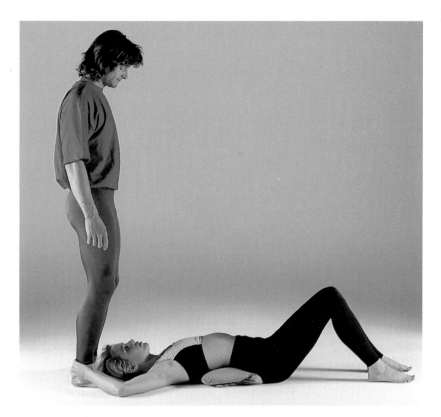

Fig. 40
Lie on your back, with your spine just above the pelvis supported from below with a roll. With both hands, grasp the ankles of your partner standing by your head, and bend your legs.

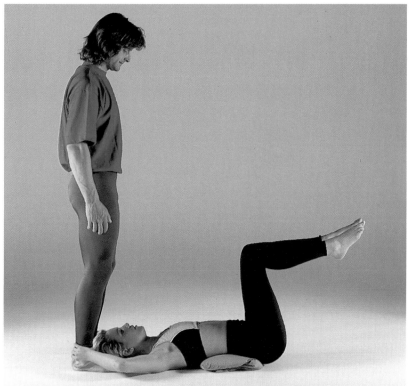

Fig. 41
With the raising of your pelvis, your hip and knee joints are flexed slowly until they are at right angles. The lumbar spine remains pressed against the roll.

Fig. 42
Sitting upright with both hands holding one knee, draw your thigh as close as possible to your torso.

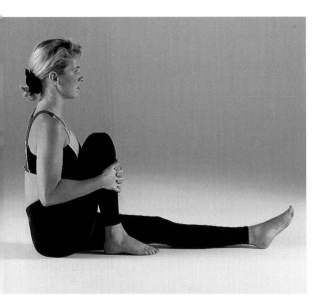

Exercises Aimed at Straightening the Spine

The exercises suggested on this and the next page require a combination of mobility and equilibrium. They are not so much aimed at strengthening the spine, as were the previous exercises, as straightening it.

Exercise

In a sitting position, clasp one leg with both hands and draw it as close as possible to your torso. Your other leg remains extended on the floor. Keep the spine as straight as you can with the strong pull on the bent leg. From this position, lower the torso, vertebra by vertebra, onto the floor, keeping the bent leg close to the torso. This exercise should be executed very slowly, and the upper torso must not suddenly fall back.

Fig. 43
Begin by leaning backward with your pelvis. Then lower your spine, vertebra by vertebra, onto the floor.

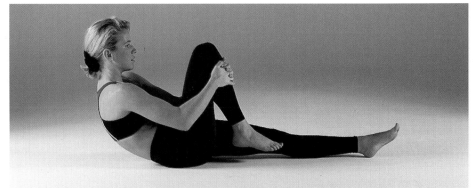

Fig. 44
How not to do it: The entire movement must be deliberate. Avoid letting the upper torso simply fall back.

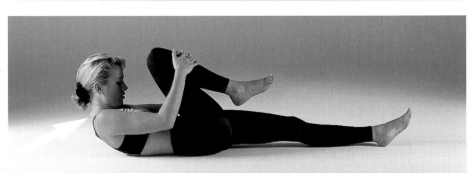

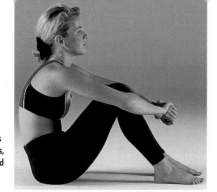

Fig. 45
Sit with both arms around your knees, your legs bent, and your feet flat on the floor.

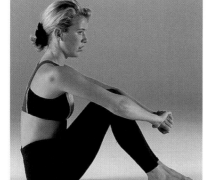

Fig. 46
Through the pull of your arms on your knees, the thoracic spine is straightened.

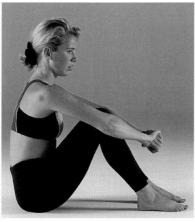

Fig. 47
The straightening effect is increased by straining upward with your head, the skin of the neck being pulled taut, while your eyes look straight ahead.

Exercise

In a sitting position with both legs bent, and your feet flat on the floor, rest your bent elbows on your knees. Then pull with your arms on the knees so that your spine is straightened, which should give you the feeling of growing taller. Without moving your eyes, strain upward with your head, causing the skin of your neck to become taut.

Exercise

Another way of working on straightening the thoracic spine in particular is to lie on a hard foam roll or a tightly rolled-up mat (see Fig. 48).

The restrictions mentioned on page 27 also apply here.

You can remain in this position as long as it is comfortable. But it should be followed by toning exercises for the abdominal and back muscles.

Fig. 48
Lie on your back, with the spine supported directly below the shoulder blades with a rolled-up mat. Stretch out your arms on the floor beyond your head.

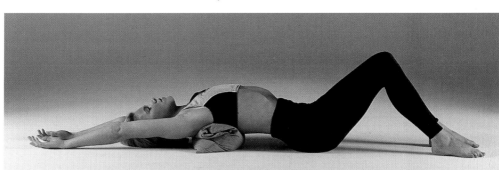

Strengthening the Back Muscles

In performing all the exercises designed to strengthen the back, take care not to "hollow" your back. Hence, you should avoid large, sweeping movements.

Exercise

For the first exercise, lie on your stomach and extend your arms beyond your head. Then tense the abdominal muscles, feeling as though a small hollow is being formed under the stomach.

You should also draw your buttocks tightly together. Keeping these muscles taut, turn the palms of your hands upward as if holding a large tray, and raise your extended arms off the floor. Your eyes are fixed on the floor.

Fig. 49
Lie on your stomach, and extend both arms beyond your head.

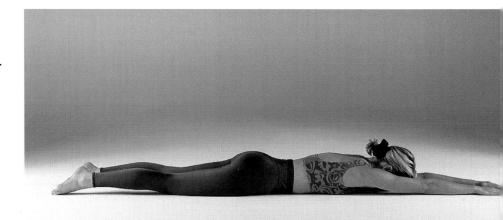

Fig. 50
With the abdominal muscles tensed, raise your extended arms. Keep your eyes fixed on the floor.

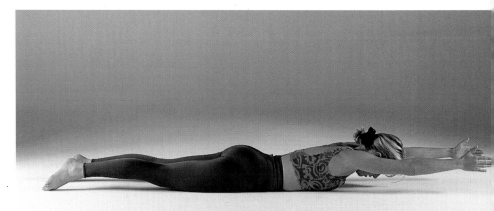

Variation

This exercise can be varied by placing
your arms behind your neck. After the
abdominal and buttock muscles have
been tensed as before, raise your
elbows so that the skin between the
shoulder blades forms a furrow.

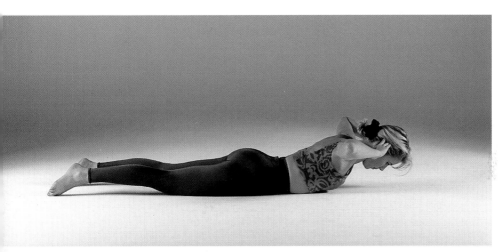

Fig. 51
**Place your hands
behind your neck,
and raise your
elbows. Keep your
eyes fixed on the
ground.**

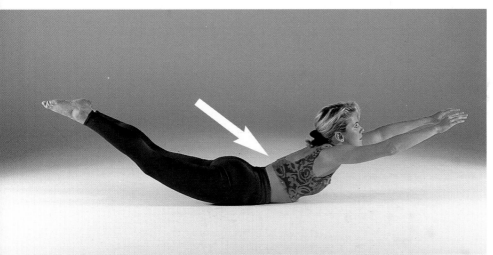

Fig. 52
**How not to do it:
In this version, the
lumbar spine is
being stretched
too much and thus
subjected to heavy
strain.**

Important Note

Fig. 52 shows an incorrect position that
strains the lumbar spine, leading to
overstretching.

Strengthening the Back Muscles with a Slight Prestretch

By using a roll of foam material or a tightly rolled-up mat, the starting position can be altered. This support should be positioned under the abdomen in such a way that it doesn't create an uncomfortable feeling of pressure.

Fig. 53
Lie on your stomach, and extend both arms beyond your head. The abdomen is supported with a roll.

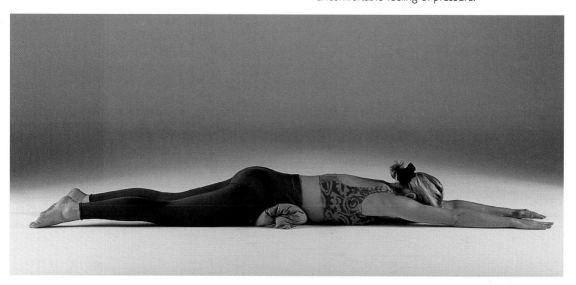

Fig. 54
Bend your legs at the knees, and lift them just an inch or two off the floor.

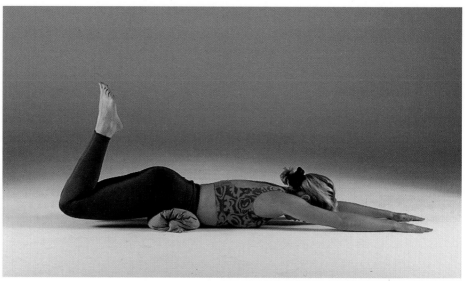

Again, extend your arms beyond your head, with your eyes fixed on the floor. First, bend your knees until the soles of your feet face toward the ceiling.

From this position, your thighs are lifted only a short distance off the floor so that you can still hold the lumbar spine straight.

Using the same starting position, keep your legs extended and lift your arms or elbows off the floor. Keep your eyes fixed on the floor, as in all the other exercises.

Fig. 55
From the prone position with the abdomen supported, raise your extended arms.

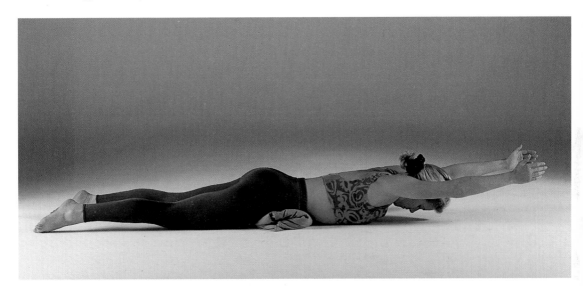

Fig. 56
From the prone position with the abdomen supported, lift your elbows upward, with your hands placed behind your neck.

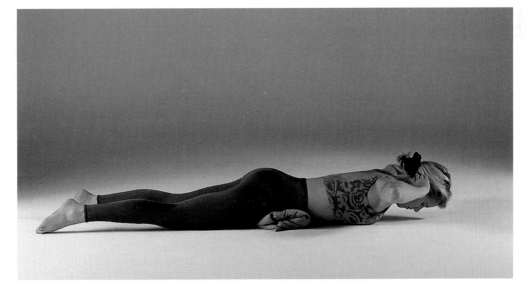

Advanced Exercise

A more difficult exercise starts with the following position: Sitting on your heels, rest your upper torso on your thighs, with your hands supported on the floor in front of your head. As you raise your torso, stretch out your arms to form an extension of the spine.

Fig. 57

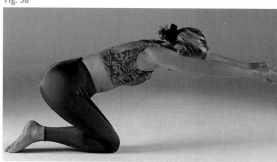

Fig. 59

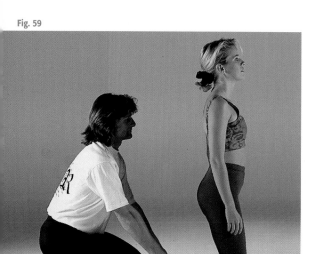

Fig. 58

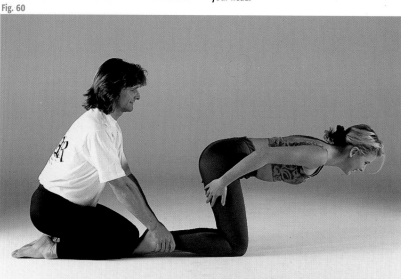

Fig. 57
Sitting on your heels, lower your upper torso until it touches your thighs, with your hands supported on the floor in front of your head.

Fig. 58
Raise your torso until it is horizontal.

Fig. 59
In the kneeling position, your feet are held down by your partner.

Fig. 60

Fig. 60
Lower your torso toward the floor, keeping your spine straight.

Working with a Partner, and a Variation

The final position often cannot be held. This is when it is useful to have the help of a partner.

In this case, your ankles are held by your partner, while you slowly lower your torso. You should continue the exercise only so long as the spine can be kept straight.

This form of the exercise can also be varied by twisting the torso from side to side.

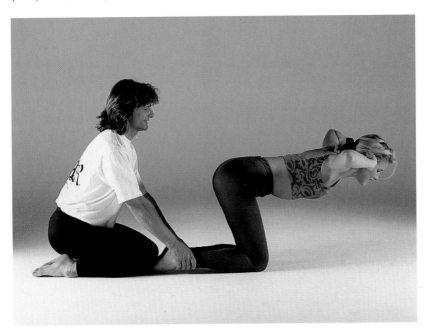

Fig. 61
In the more difficult form of the exercise, you place your hands at the back of your head.

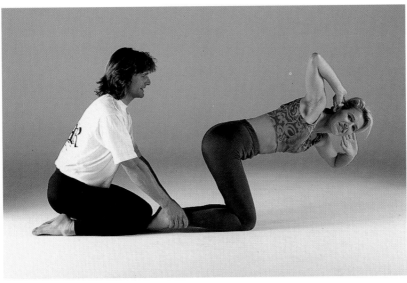

Fig. 62
In the variation of the exercise, you twist your torso alternately to the right and the left, with your head following the movement.

If you find the starting position too difficult because of problems with your knees, then the prone position should be used.

Here, again, take care not to compensate by hollowing the back.

Exercise

To start in a more secure position, bend one leg at the hip and the knee sideways from the body. But this position must be comfortable, because you will need to relax briefly in it during the break between repetitions of the exercise. The variations are the same as with the previous two exercises.

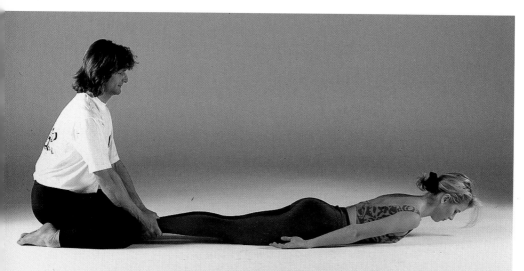

Fig. 63
Lie on your stomach, with your feet held by your partner. Raise your head and shoulders slightly off the floor. Fix your eyes on the floor and stretch your neck.

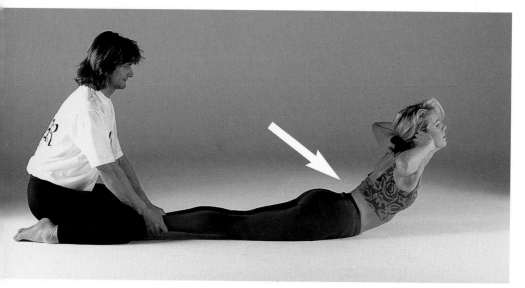

Fig. 64
How not to do it: Here, the lumbar spine is being stretched too much, causing possible adverse strain.

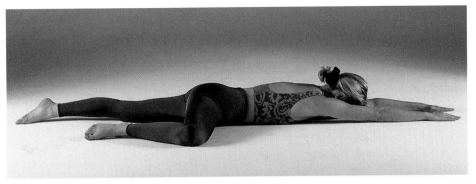

Fig. 65
Lie on your stomach, bending one leg sideways from your body. Stretch out your arms straight in front of your head.

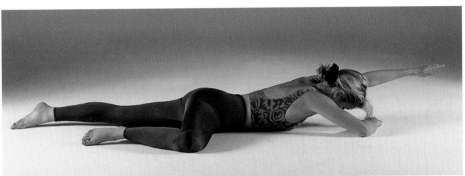

Fig. 66
While pressing hard on the floor with one arm, raise the other one, still extended. Keep your eyes fixed on the floor.

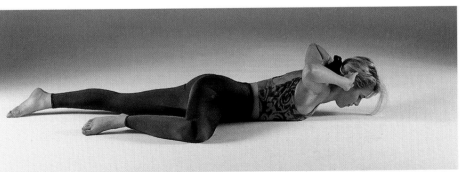

Fig. 67
Lift both arms off the floor at the same time, and raise them to shoulder height, keeping your eyes fixed on the floor.

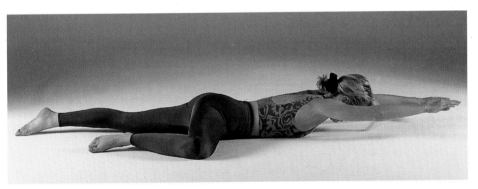

Fig. 68
In the more difficult version, you place your hands on the back of your head and lift your elbows upward, keeping your eyes fixed on the floor.

Mobilization of the Spine

The following exercise is designed to improve mobility rather than strength.

Sitting on your heels, lower your torso onto your thighs, while your hands rest on the floor beyond your head. While the hand of one arm presses hard on the floor, the other arm is lifted, still extended, toward the ceiling.

Keep your eyes fixed on the palm of your raised hand, and turn your head following the arm as far as possible in the same direction.

You should maintain the tension on the opposite side throughout the exercise.

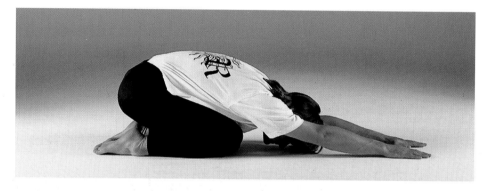

Fig. 69
Sitting on your heels, lower your torso until it touches your thighs. Your arms are extended in front of your head, with the palms of your hands resting on the floor.

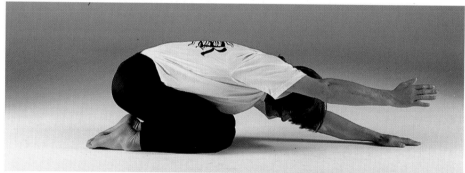

Fig. 70
While pressing on the floor with one hand, raise the other toward the ceiling. Allow your torso to lift only slightly off your thighs.

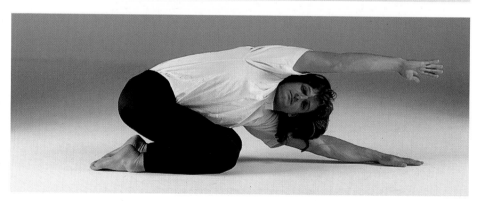

Fig. 71
A variation of the exercise: You fix your eyes on the palm of your raised hand, and your head follows the movement.

Strengthening the Stabilizing Muscles of the Pelvis and the Trunk

The following exercises are aimed at groups of muscles that are often neglected.

These exercises are just as important for stabilizing the pelvic and torso muscles as the abdominal and back muscles.

In some of the exercises, the muscles involved can on occasion develop a cramp. If this occurs, the exercise should be stopped and not repeated the same day. Experience shows that this effect disappears as you become more proficient in exercising. But should cramping persist, it is wise to consult an expert (such as a medical practitioner) to find the cause of the problem.

As with the toning exercises for the back muscles, it is important that no compensatory movements be made. These are described separately in each case.

Exercise

Lie on your side with your legs together, and one hand supported on the floor in front of your chest. The upper arm can then stabilize your upper torso. Raise the upper leg not more than about 40 degrees. Follow with the lower leg, bringing it as close as possible to the upper leg. Meanwhile, the pelvis must not twist back, as is clearly shown in the wrong version (Fig. 75).

Fig. 74
Follow with the lower leg, raising it as close as possible to the upper leg.

Fig. 75
How not to do it: The upper part of the pelvis twists, and the position cannot be stabilized.

If you find it difficult to do the exercise, then don't raise the top leg so high. Once you feel confident doing this exercise, you can dispense with the supporting hand.

Fig. 72
Lie on your side, with your body stretched out straight. Place your upper hand on the floor in front of your chest for support.

Fig. 73
Raise the upper leg.

Fig. 72

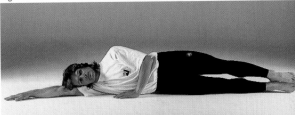

Fig. 73

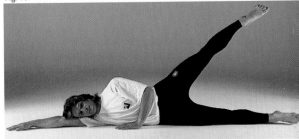

Fig. 74

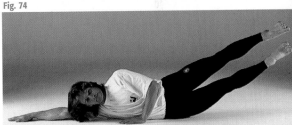

Fig. 75

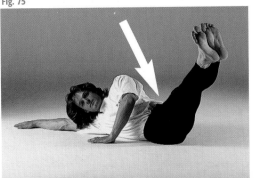

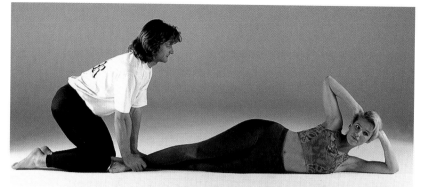

Fig. 76
Lie on one side
with your legs
slightly apart a
if taking a step,
your feet held
your partner, a
your hands
placed on the
back of your
head.

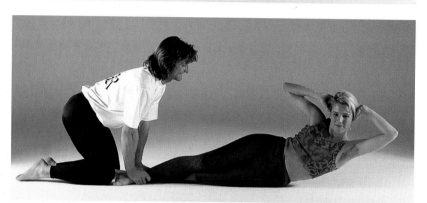

Fig. 77
Raise your
upper torso,
bending
sideways.

Fig. 78
A variation of the
exercise: You turn
your lower shoulder
upward, and your
eyes look toward
your partner.

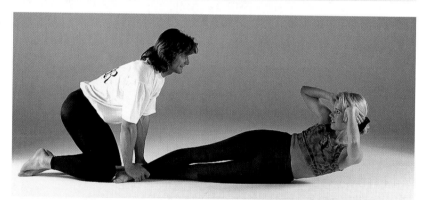

Fig. 79
How not to do it:
The upper part of
the pelvis twists,
and the position
cannot be stabilized.

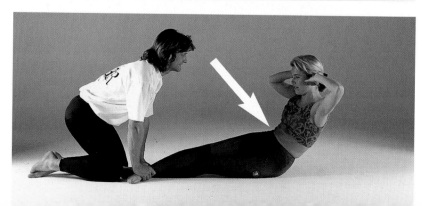

Working with a Partner

In this exercise your partner again has to secure the starting position.

Lie on one side, with your legs slightly apart as if taking a step, and the knee of your upper leg slightly bent. From this position, raise your body sideways. It is not possible to move very far, and it is also unnecessary for the correct execution of the exercise.

Variations

The illustrations show the more difficult form of the exercise with the hands on the back of the head. If you hold your arms parallel to your body, the exercise is easier. You can vary the exercise by turning your upper body and looking at your partner.

Important Note

It would be a mistake to twist the pelvis and raise yourself by bending at the hips, because this doesn't involve the desired muscle group.

Exercise

Lie on one side, with your torso supported by the lower arm that rests on the floor. Its elbow should be below the shoulder joint. You can rest the hand of the top arm in front of your chest on the floor as an aid for balance when the pelvis is lifted. Your entire body should be in a straight line and completely taut.

Fig. 80
Lying on your side, support yourself on your lower arm, with the hand from the other arm placed in front of you on the floor.

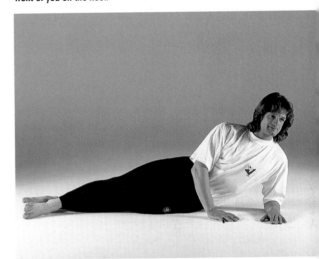

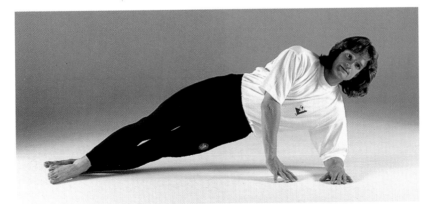

Fig. 81
Lift your pelvis until your entire body is in a straight line. The hand resting on the floor acts as a support for the movement.

Advanced Version

Given sufficient strength at the outset, you can dispense with support from the upper arm. And if the body is in excellent equilibrium, the upper leg can be raised, as well. But take care that the upper part of your pelvis doesn't twist back.

Variation

The exercise can be varied further by placing the palm of the hand on the floor as support, but this is only recommended if you have strong wrists. Make sure that the elbow is slightly bent so that the elbow joint is held secure by the muscle tension.

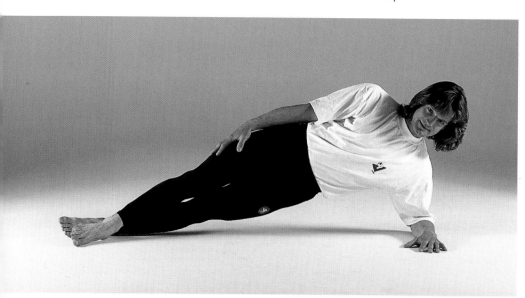

Fig. 82
Without the support of the hand of the upper arm, the exercise becomes more difficult.

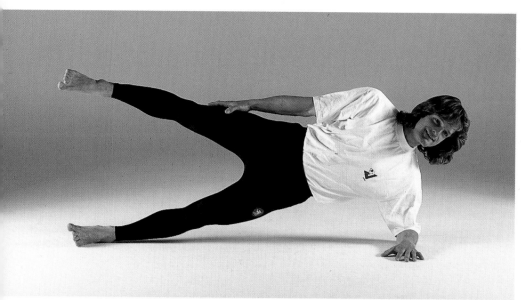

Fig. 83
By raising the upper leg, the exercise can be made even harder.

Be Careful!
With the elbow straightened, the active support of the muscles disappears. The joints are only held in place by the ligaments.

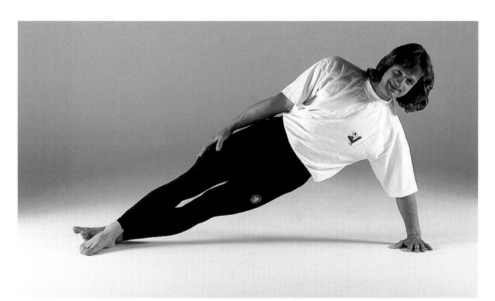

Fig. 84
In a one-handed sideways push-up, bring your body into a straight line. Keep the elbow of the supporting arm bent slightly.

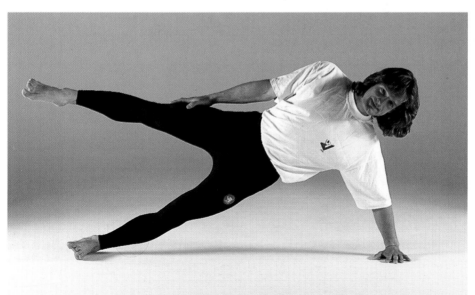

Fig. 85
In the more difficult version of the exercise, you raise the upper leg.

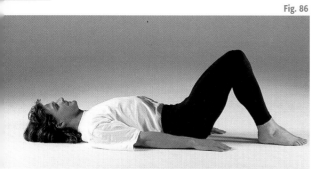

Fig. 86

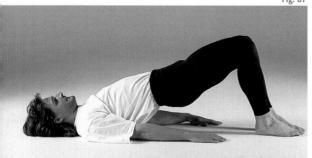

Fig. 87

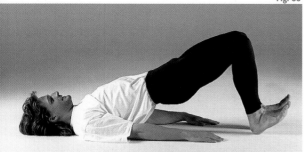

Fig. 88

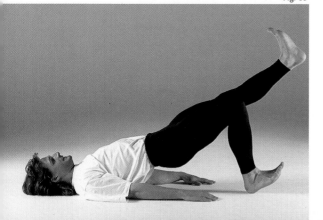

Fig. 89

Exercise

Another exercise involving the muscles of the pelvis and the trunk starts from a supine position. Bend both legs with your feet on the floor, and your hands resting beside the buttocks. First press the lumbar vertebrae against the floor with the help of the abdominal muscles. Then lift your pelvis off the floor until your thighs and torso are in a straight line.

By pulling the tips of your toes strongly upward toward the shins, the tension can be increased.

Fig. 86
Lie on your back with your legs bent, and your hands resting beside the buttocks.

Fig. 87
Raise your pelvis to form a straight-line extension of your thighs and torso.

Fig. 88
In the raised position, pull the tips of the toes of both feet strongly upward.

Fig. 89
Raise one leg to form a straight line with your torso, pull the tips of the toes strongly upward, and push the heel away from your body.

Advanced Version

If, in addition, you raise one leg and make it also form a straight line with your torso, then the exercise is even more effective. Again, take care that the hip of the straightened leg doesn't drop as a possible compensatory movement.

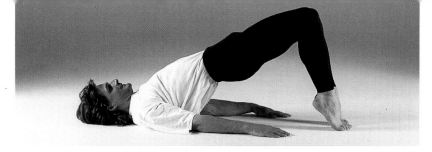

Fig. 90
In the raised position, rest the tips of your toes on the floor.

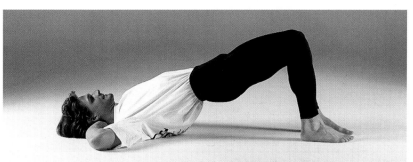

Fig. 91
In the raised position with your feet flat on the floor, place both hands under your head. Press hard with your elbows against the floor.

Variation

Instead of pulling the tips of your toes upward toward the shins, you can point them down to rest on the floor. This produces extreme tensing of the small muscles of the foot. This muscle group is generally underused in everyday life, and is easily overstrained in this exercise, leading to an increased liability to cramp. However, experience indicates that the tendency to cramp soon disappears as you become more proficient in exercising (see page 41).

A further variation of this exercise is executed with the arms folded and the hands under your head. Supported on both legs or in the more difficult form on only one leg, you press hard against the floor with your forearms and your elbows.

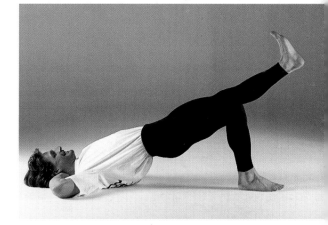

Fig. 92
Raise one leg to form a straight extension of the torso; then strongly pull the tips of the toes of both feet upward.

Fig. 93
How not to do it: One side of the pelvis drops down.

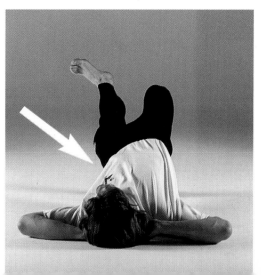

Exercise

For the following exercise, excellent stabilizing ability is required, so you must master the previous exercises first.

Advanced Version

Sitting with your legs bent, support yourself on the floor with your fists, bending your elbows slightly. Lift the pelvis off the floor, and raise it until the thighs form a straight line with the torso.

Your elbows should remain bent slightly, and your torso should not drop down between the supporting arms.

Even greater stability is required when, as in previous exercises, one leg is lifted to form an extension of the torso.

This is a difficult exercise, which should be attempted only if you are in excellent shape.

Fig. 94
Sit on the floor with your legs bent, and your hands forming fists and resting on the floor, with the elbows bent slightly.

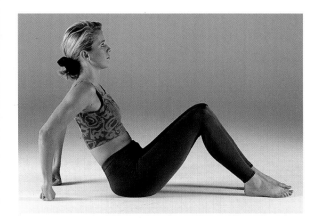

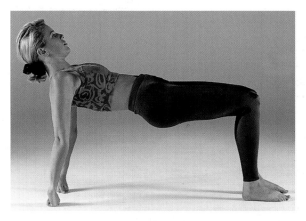

Fig. 95
Raise your pelvis to form a straight line with the torso and the thighs. Keep your elbows bent slightly.

Fig. 96
Raise one leg to form a straight extension of the torso, and strongly pull the tips of your toes upward.

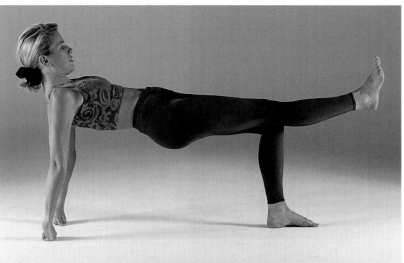

Strengthening the Stabilizing Muscles of the Shoulder Girdle and the Trunk

The shoulders have already been worked on in some of the previous exercises. The exercises on the next few pages again are shown at different levels of difficulty with some possible variations. However, first a test of the stabilizing ability of the shoulder girdle will be described. If weaknesses are revealed from the test, begin with simple exercises, as discussed on page 14.

Test of the Stabilizing Ability of the Shoulder Girdle

The shoulders' stabilizing muscles are often not as strong as they should be. The test suggested here gives you a general idea of their state.

Test (Fig. 97)

Kneel on the floor in a "bench position," resting on your forearms. With tensed abdominal muscles, slowly shift the weight of your torso forward over the supporting forearms.

During this maneuver, keep your spine straight and don't let your torso drop between your arms (Fig. 98). If there is a lack of stability, after a few seconds of holding this position one shoulder blade or both may move out of position, or your torso may also drop down between your upper arms.

Note
This test can also be used as a strengthening exercise for the muscle groups concerned.

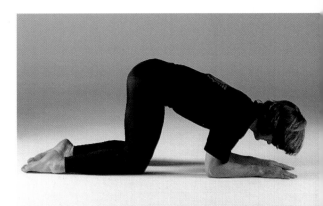

Fig. 97
Testing the stabilizing ability of the shoulder girdle:
Supporting yourself on your calves and your forearms, slowly shift the weight of your torso forward. Keep your spine as straight as possible, and do not let your upper body drop between the supporting arms.

Fig. 98
Lack of stabilizing ability in the shoulder girdle:
After a short while, you lose the stable position. The spine and the trunk sink down into a compensating position.

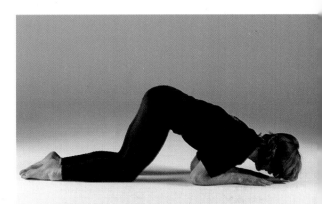

Exercise

The "bench position" (kneeling on the floor, resting on the hands) provides an easy-to-control way of putting pressure on the muscles of your shoulder girdle. You support your weight either on the palms of your hands or, if the wrists are weak, on your fists.

Place your hands directly below the shoulder joints. In the starting position, open your knees in line with your hips, and rest your feet either on the instep or the toes.

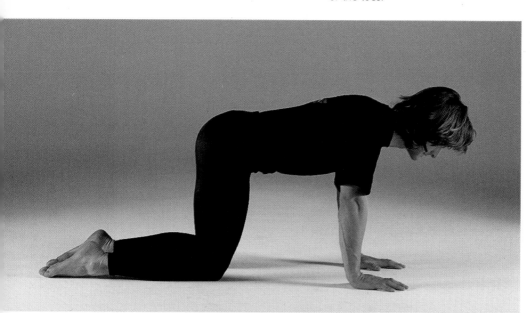

Fig. 99
Support yourself on your insteps, knees, and hands, with your elbows bent slightly. Keep your spine as straight as possible.

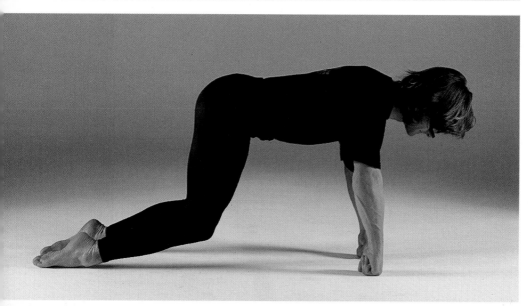

Fig. 100
By pressing on the floor with your insteps, you take the weight off your knees, which are lifted slightly. Keep your elbows slightly bent.

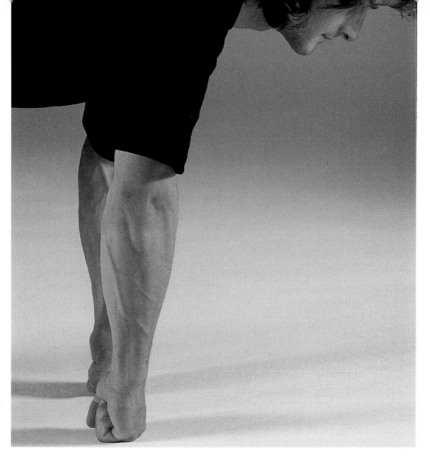

Fig. 101
If your wrists are weak, then form fists and use them as support instead of your palms.

Fig. 102
If you have difficulties with your ankle joints, then switch support from the insteps to the toes.

At the start of the exercise, take the weight off your knees by pressing hard with your feet on the floor. Here, a couple of inches between the knees and the floor are enough. As in all support exercises, keep the elbows bent slightly.

You can control the intensity of this exercise by shifting your weight into a different position over your supporting hands. Your personal load limit is reached when your shoulders begin to drop down between the supporting arms.

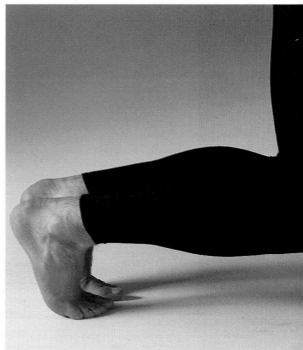

Advanced Version

If you can hold a position in which the torso remains far forward over the hands without effort for several seconds, you should reduce the amount of support. You can do this by lifting a leg, or an arm, or a leg and the arm of the opposite side (Figs. 103 and 104).

Further Increasing the Load

The classic push-up can be used very successfully as one of the shoulder girdle stabilizing exercises.

Here, again, it is often necessary to return to the exercises on the previous pages if the required final position cannot be held correctly.

Another preliminary exercise requires the forearms to be used as support (Fig. 105). In this case, you should keep the body taut, so that the lumbar spine and the torso do not sag between the upper arms (Fig.106). You can again rest your feet either on the insteps or the toes.

Note

If, in addition, you lift a leg off the floor, this must not lead to the compensating movement shown in Fig. 108, as this again overstretches the lumbar spine.

Fig. 103
In the more difficult version, you lift one foot off the floor.

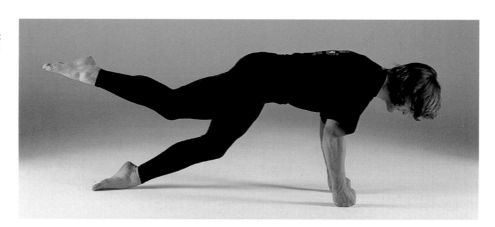

Fig. 104
The exercise is further intensified if you lift one hand off the floor, as well.

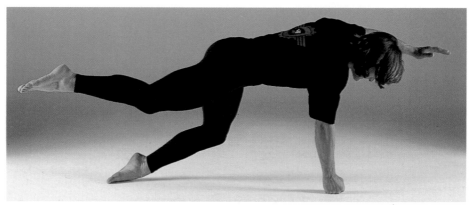

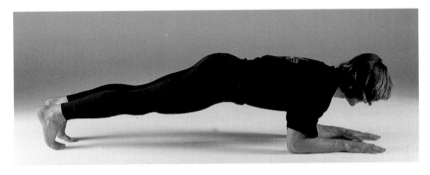

Fig. 105
In the push-up
position resting
on the forearms,
make your body
as taut as
possible.

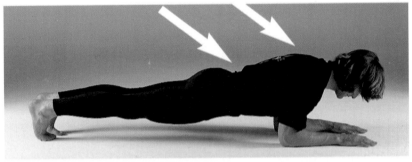

Fig. 106
How not to do it:
The lumbar spine
sags, so the
shoulder girdle
cannot be
stabilized.

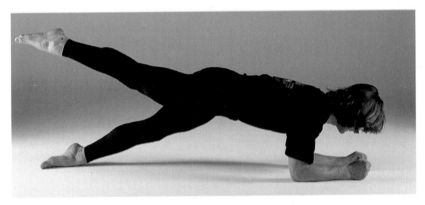

Fig. 107
In the more
advanced exercise,
you lift one leg off
the floor.

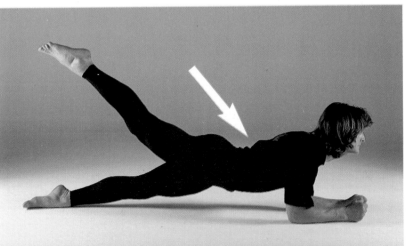

Fig. 108
How not to do it:
Raising your leg
should not lead to
any compensating
movement.

Exercise

Sometimes supporting yourself on the forearms seems more difficult than the push-up position where you are resting on your hands, although the lower-arm support is considered a preliminary exercise. The reason is that push-ups are often done incorrectly. Your elbows should always be bent slightly in the high position. Even when the exercise consists of the up-and-down movement of the trunk, the reversal of the movement should always occur before the elbows are straightened fully.

If this proves difficult, you should at first try it in the held position—that is, without bending or straightening the arms.

Note

If a compensating movement occurs (Fig. 111), you should return to a simpler form of the exercise. Another way of correcting the error is to curve the torso.

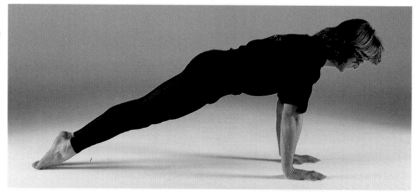

Fig. 109
In the push-up position resting on the hands, make your body as taut as possible.

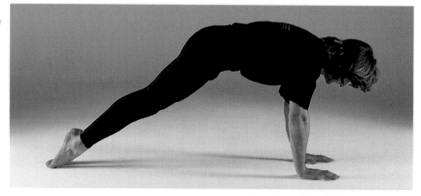

Fig. 110
If you cannot hold the stable position, you should round your back.

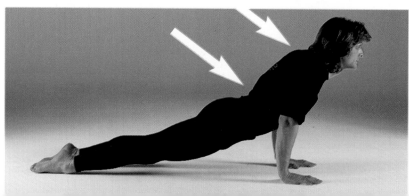

Fig. 111
How not to do it:
The pelvis and the lumbar spine sag—hence, the shoulders cannot be stabilized.

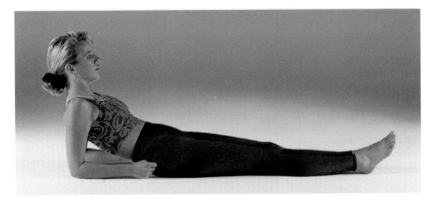

Fig. 112
Partially sitting with legs straight, support the upper body with your forearms resting alongside it.

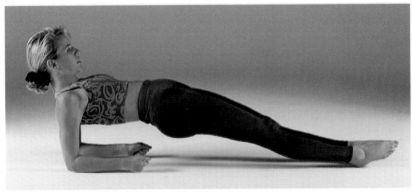

Fig. 113
Lift the pelvis until your torso and legs form a straight line.

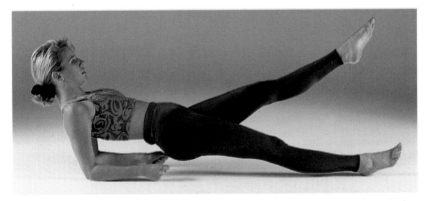

Fig. 114
In the more difficult form of the exercise, lift one leg off the floor and raise it slightly.

Exercise

Reverse push-ups can be executed in a manner similar to the support exercises that are performed from the prone position. In this position, you can easily control any undesirable compensating movements. Place your elbows so that they are below the shoulders in the support position.

Take care that your torso does not sag between the supporting arms, and that when the straightened leg is raised, the hip on that side doesn't drop.

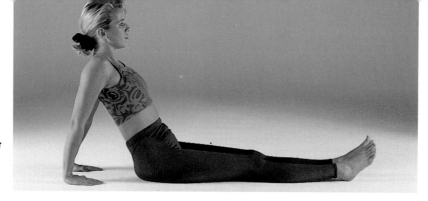

Fig. 115
In a sitting position with fully extended legs, support your upper body with your hands placed behind the buttocks. Keep your elbows bent slightly.

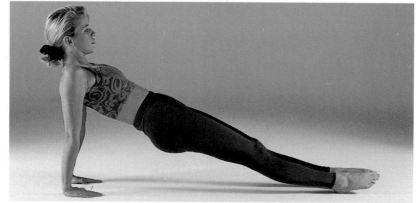

Fig. 116
Raise your pelvis until the torso and the legs form a straight line.

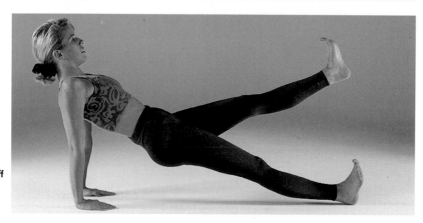

Fig. 117
In the more difficult version, lift one leg off the floor and raise it in the air.

Advanced Version

As before, you can increase the load by reducing the support surface. However, if you get a pain in the wrists when using the hand support, then the fists should be used instead.

Reminders

In all support exercises, keep your elbows bent slightly.

When raising the straightened leg, as before you must not allow the hip on that side to drop.

Advanced Version

To execute the following exercise, you must already be well stabilized throughout your entire muscle system.

In a partial sitting position with your legs bent, support the upper body with your forearms. From this position, raise your pelvis until the torso forms a straight line with the thighs. Do not allow the trunk to sag between the supporting arms.

This form of stabilization, like the exercise on page 48, should be attempted only if you are in good shape.

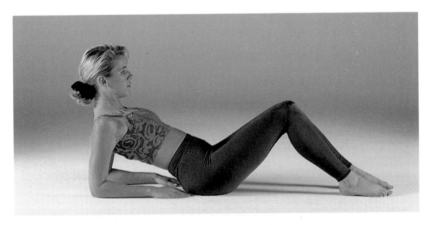

Fig. 118
In a partial sitting position with your legs bent, support the upper body with your forearms resting parallel to it.

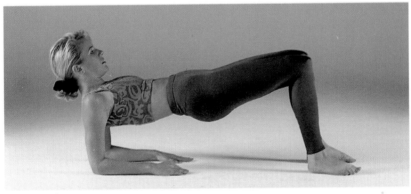

Fig. 119
Raise your pelvis until your torso and thighs form a straight line.

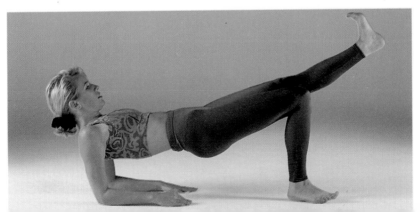

Fig. 120
In the more advanced version, raise one leg until it forms a straight line with the torso.

Strengthening the Buttock Muscles and the Lower Extensors of the Back

In all exercises that require you to lift your pelvis while lying on your back, the buttock, or gluteus, muscles are activated.

There is relatively little need for stabilization in this case. After a short description of how to test the tone of the buttock muscles, exercises follow that are aimed specifically at this group of muscles and the extensors of the back.

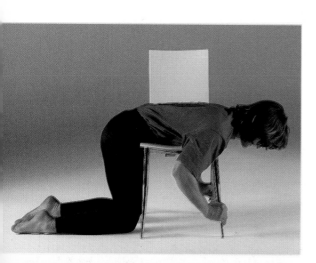

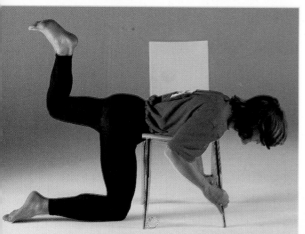

Testing the Strength of the Buttocks Muscles

The muscles of the buttocks perform an important stabilizing function for the pelvis. They are often poorly developed, as are the abdominal muscles.

Test (Figs. 121 and 122)

Lie on your stomach over a chair, which may be padded with a blanket; the pelvis must be resting on the chair, as well. Find something firm for your hands to hold on to, and bring the thighs as close to the chair as possible.

Continue to push against the chair with one thigh, while raising the other leg, which is bent at the knee, until the hip joint is straightened. If you can bring the thigh of the raised leg into the horizontal position, or straighten the hip slightly, without decreasing the pressure of the other leg against the chair, then the hip extensors are strong.

You may not be able to reach the final position due to the inability of the hip flexors to stretch. That is why they should be tested before attempting the exercise.

Note

This test is also suitable as a strengthening exercise for the relevant group of muscles.

Fig. 121
Testing the strength of the buttock muscles:
For the starting position, lie on your stomach over a padded chair so that your pelvis rests on it, as well. Hold the chair legs with your hands, and draw your thighs close to the chair.

Fig. 122
Then press hard against the chair with one thigh, while raising the other leg with the knee bent until the hip joint is straight.

Strengthening the Hip Extensors

Exercise

In the following exercise, which you execute while lying on your stomach, it is particularly important that no compensating movements occur. This is achieved by making the abdominal muscles work very hard. By forming a little hollow under the abdomen, at least in your imagination, you can protect the pelvis and the lumbar spine. Keep one leg straight, and bend the other at the knee. Then lift the bent leg; just a short distance is enough.

Advanced Version

If in the advanced form of this exercise, you lift both legs with the knees bent, it is even more important to stabilize the pelvis properly.

Always avoid hollowing the back.

This and the following exercise can sometimes cause more of a tendency for the muscles at the back of the thighs to cramp. Should you find that this is the case, the advice given on page 41 applies. Also, if you suffer cramps, under no circumstances should you repeat the exercise on the same day; instead, you should follow it up with the stretching exercise on page 69.

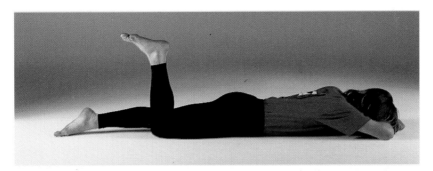

Fig. 123
Lie on your stomach, with one leg bent at the knee and your arms lying in a relaxed position.

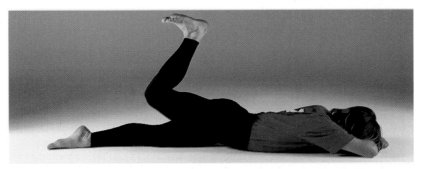

Fig. 124
Lift the thigh of the bent leg off the floor, and raise it slightly. Pull the tips of your toes strongly in the direction of the shins.

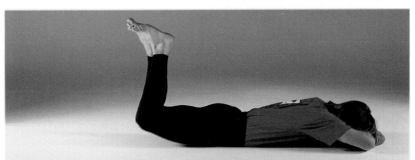

Fig. 125
In the more advanced version, you lift both legs slightly off the floor.

Variation

If the pelvis cannot be protected adequately, then the exercise can be performed from a different starting position. Lie on your stomach, with one leg bent and your torso resting on your thigh. Keep the other leg straight, and lay your hands beside your head.

Then bend the free leg at the knee, and raise it off the floor. Again, a movement of a couple of inches is sufficient to achieve a powerful tensing of the muscles. The prerequisites for the successful execution of this exercise are sufficient strength in the buttock muscles and adequate stretch in the hip flexors. Accordingly, you should first test your ability to stretch the hip flexors (see page 73). If you are unable to achieve any movement from the starting position, then it is enough for a start to hold the position with the muscles tensed.

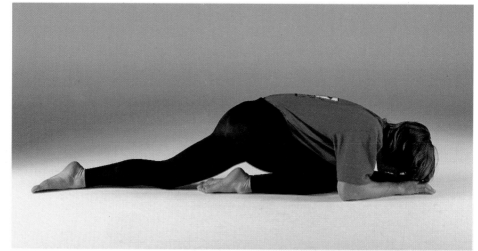

Fig. 126
Lie on your stomach, with one leg pulled up under your torso, keeping the other one straight. Rest your torso on the thigh of the bent leg.

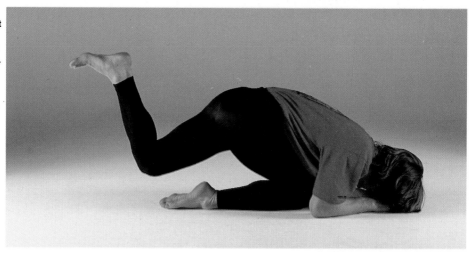

Fig. 127
Bend the straight leg at the knee, and lift it slightly. Keep the torso in the starting position.

Advanced Version

If you are able to perform the exercise test as a result of having a well-stabilized pelvis, the exercise can be intensified by also raising the arm diagonally opposite. All the previous instructions apply. (Note: The photos show both arms.)

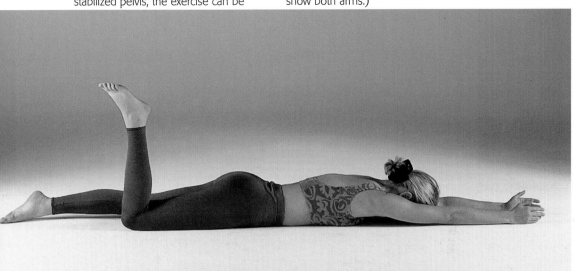

Fig. 128
Lie on your stomach, with one leg bent at the knee. Rest the arm on the opposite side fully extended on the floor.

Fig. 129
Lift the bent leg and the fully extended arm off the floor at the same time, and raise them slightly.

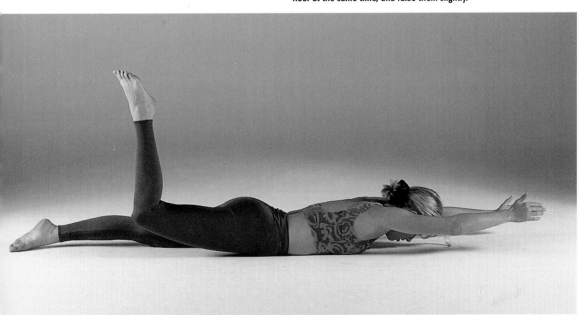

Strengthening the Extensors of the Back, Starting with a Slight Prestretch

A workout aimed specifically at the lower sections of the extensors of the back can be achieved with the aid of a chair and a roll of firm foam or a tightly rolled-up mat.

Lie facedown over a chair, and place the roll under your body so that the lumbar spine is rounded slightly.

When your hands have a firm grip on the legs of the chair, lift your knees and your calves off the floor and raise the pelvis until the spine is straight.

Repeat the exercise several times, without putting your knees and calves on the floor.

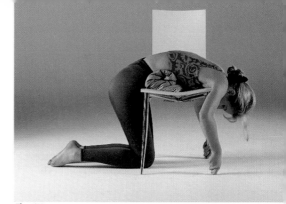

Fig. 130

Fig,

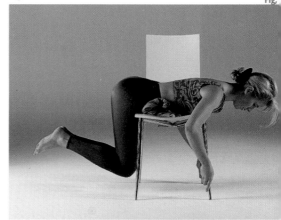

Fig. 132
Lie on your back, with one leg bent, its foot on the floor. Clasp the knee of your other leg with both hands. Now pull the thigh of your bent leg close to your torso.

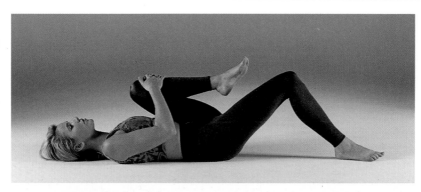

Fig. 130
Lie facedown o a chair, with yo trunk supporte just above the pelvis with a rc Bend your knee and hips.

Fig. 131
Lift your calves the floor, and r them until the spine is straigh

Fig. 133
Raise the pelvis until your torso and thigh are in a straight line. Keep the bent leg you are clasping in contact with the torso.

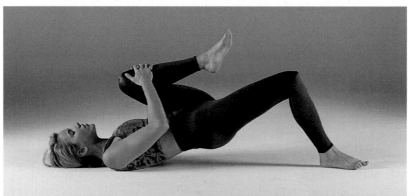

Examples of Combined Exercises

Before concluding the section on toning, or strengthening, exercises, a few exercises made up of combinations of different elements from the previous pages will be described.

You should attempt these routines only when you have mastered the simpler exercises and your mobility has improved.

Advanced Exercises

Lie on your back, clasping one knee with both hands and pulling it close to your chest. Bend the other leg at the knee, and rest the sole of its foot on the floor. By pressing hard on the supporting leg, lift your pelvis so that as straight a line as possible is formed by your torso and thigh. The leg you have pulled up should move only a little away from your body.

Again, lying on your back, bend one leg back until the knee meets the palm of your hand on the same side. Keep the other leg bent with the foot on the floor as before, while the arm on that side lies alongside your buttock.

First, press hard with your hand against the bent back knee, pushing the knee toward the palm at the same time. When you can feel the tensing of the abdominal muscles, your pelvis will be raised until the torso and the thigh are again in a straight line due to the pressure on the supporting leg. You can also exert downward pressure with the hand resting on the floor.

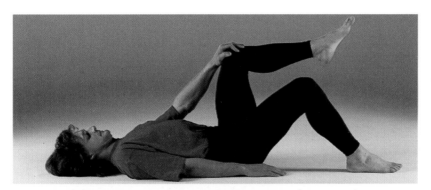

Fig. 134
Lie on your back, with one leg bent and the foot on the floor, and then bend the other leg back until the knee meets the palm of your hand on that side.

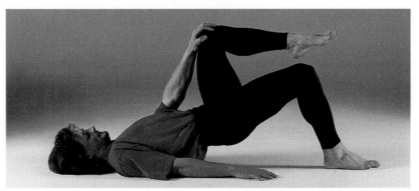

Fig. 135
While you press with your hand against the bent back knee, push the knee against the hand. Your pelvis is raised until the torso and the thigh form a straight line.

Variations

In a variation of the previous exercise that has a greater effect on the shoulder girdle, bend one arm and place it above your head. Tension is created by the strong pressure of the lower arm and the elbow.

A powerful effort is required of the abdominal muscles in the following stabilization exercise from a supine position. Bend both arms and rest them above your head, while you draw both legs toward your torso. Keep the lumbar spine pressed against the floor, and maintain this position during the ensuing movement of the legs.

Bend and extend each of your legs in turn parallel to the floor, tensing the muscles of your extended leg by pulling hard on the tips of your toes.

You can increase the effect of the last exercise on the abdominal muscles by lifting your head and pushing your hands in the direction of your heels. The leg movement remains as before.

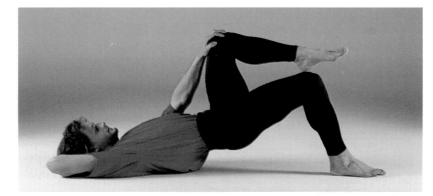

Fig. 136
A variation of the exercise: Rest one arm above your head, while pressing hard with the elbow and the lower arm against the floor.

Fig. 137
Lie on your back, with both arms reaching beyond your head. With tensed abdominal muscles, bend and extend each of your legs in turn just above the floor.

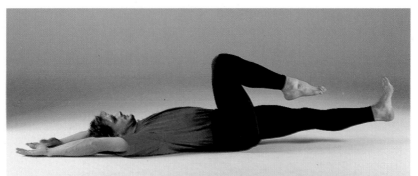

Fig. 138
In the more difficult version, you also raise your head, with your eyes fixed on your knees. Push your hands in the direction of your heels.

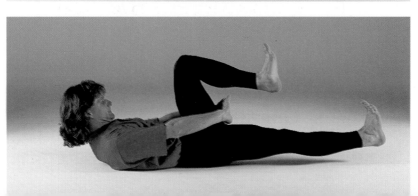

Exercises to Improve Mobility

The exercises presented here for improving mobility are mainly specific stretching positions, apart from a few general mobilization exercises. For recommendations regarding how to execute stretching exercises, refer to the guidelines on page 13.

Tests to ascertain the stretching ability of important muscle groups always precede the relevant mobility exercises. Each of these test positions can itself be used as a stretching position, or exercise. Testing the stretching ability of the muscles of the spine is not attempted here, because this is not a check you can make on yourself.

Stretching the Calves

Certain muscle groups have a tendency to lose stretching ability, and the calf muscles are one of them, especially the deeper muscle layers.

Tests for the Stretching Ability of the Calf Muscles

Test

If you can reach the floor from a low crouching position only by lifting your heels off the floor, then your calf muscles may have shortened (Fig. 139). Because tall people are at a disadvantage when they try this test, it's important to bear in mind the limitations that apply to test positions.

Your stretching ability is satisfactory if you can easily achieve the low crouching position (Fig. 140).

Test

Employing the upper layer of the calf muscles, you should be able to raise your foot at least enough to form a right angle while keeping your knee straight (Fig. 141). If you feel undue strain in the calf, this can be a sign of a lack of stretching ability.

Fig. 139
Lack of stretching ability in the deeper layers of the calf muscles: **Here, the low crouching position has only been achieved with the heels raised, but the limitations already mentioned must be taken into account.**

Fig. 140
Satisfactory stretching ability in the deeper layers of the calf muscles: **The low crouching position can easily be achieved.**

Fig. 141
Testing the stretching ability of the upper layer of the calf muscles: **Sitting on the floor with one leg bent and one straight, pull the foot of the straight leg strongly toward the body.**

Fig. 141
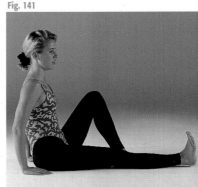

139
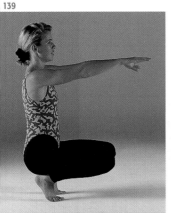

Fig. 140
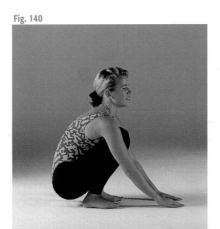

Exercises

Targeted stretching of the calf muscles is achieved with two complementary exercises. For these, it's advisable to hold onto a chair or support yourself against a wall.

Assume a position for taking a stride, with the toes of both feet pointing forward, and then transfer your weight to the front leg. Keep the heel of the back foot on the floor, while slowly straightening the knee of the back leg until you can feel the stretching of the calf muscles.

The second version is done from the same starting position, only the stride you take is somewhat shorter. Bend the knee of the back leg as far as you can without raising the heel.

This position is not always felt to be a stretch; this shouldn't, however, cause you to abandon it.

Intensified Stretching

The first two stretches can be intensified by placing the front third of the foot on a book or something similar. Do the exercises as before, taking even greater care that the heel of the back leg remains on the floor.

Important Note

Fig. 148 shows an incorrect exercise that is frequently used as a stretch for the calf muscles. Performing this exercise only makes sense when there is already excellent stretching ability in the calf muscles. In most cases, however, it simply strains the lumbar spine.

Fig. 142

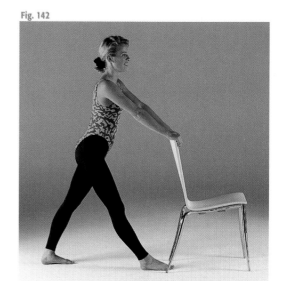

Fig. 143

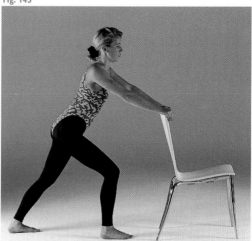

Fig. 144

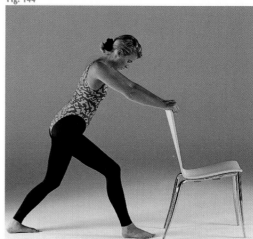

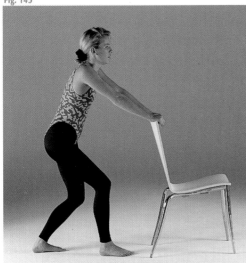

Fig. 145

Fig. 142
Take up a stride position, with both hands resting on a chair and the toes of both feet pointing forward.

Fig. 143
Shift your weight onto the front foot, and straighten the knee of the back leg. Keep the heel of the back foot on the floor.

Fig. 144
In the stride position, bend the knee of the back leg slightly.

Fig. 145
Further increase the bending of the back knee, without lifting the heel of the back foot off the floor.

Figs. 146 and 147
You can intensify the stretching in the last two exercises if you rest the front part of the foot on a book.

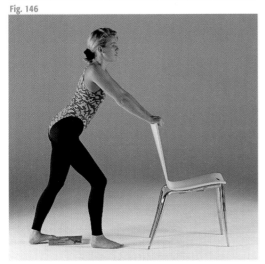

Fig. 146

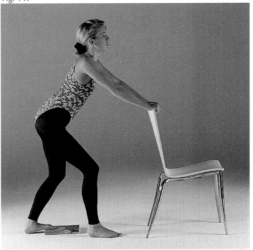

Fig. 147

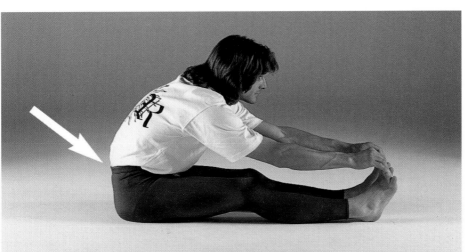

Fig. 148
How not to do it: When the calf muscles are shortened, this stretch exercise strains the lumbar spine.

Stretching the Back of the Thighs

The muscles in the back of the thighs often also have a reduced stretching ability.

Testing the Stretching Ability of the Muscles in the Back of the Thighs

Test

Lie on your back, holding one leg with both hands at the back of the knee. Straighten the other leg, and press it against the floor. Straighten also the raised leg at the knee, and flex it as far as possible in the hip. Good stretching ability is demonstrated if you can achieve the final position shown in Fig. 149.

It must be assumed that stretching ability is reduced if, with your knee straight, the flexing at the hip is appreciably less than 90 degrees.

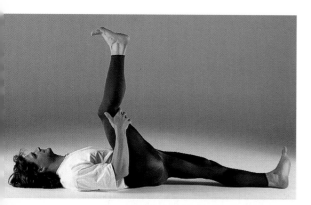

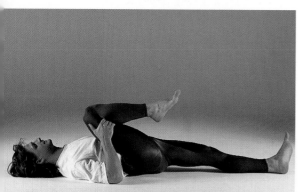

Fig. 149
Testing the stretching ability of the muscles in the back of the thighs: **Lie on your back, holding one leg with both hands at the back of the knee, which is straight, while pressing the other leg against the floor. Pull the raised leg toward your torso as far as possible.**

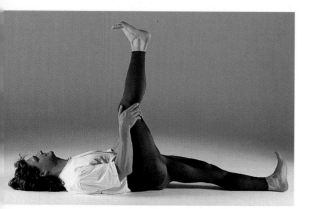

Fig. 150
Lie on your back, and grasp the back of the knee of one leg with both hands, while keeping the other leg straight. Pull the thigh toward the torso.

Fig. 151
Slowly straighten the knee of the bent leg. Meanwhile, maintain the flexing of the hip.

Exercise

Lie on your back, holding one leg with both hands at the back of the knee, and keeping the other leg fully extended on the floor. With both hands, pull the thigh as close as possible to the torso.

Maintain the considerable flexing of the hip, while slowly straightening the knee of the bent leg.

Variation

You can also transfer the stretching to the calf muscles by pulling the tips of the toes strongly in the direction of the shin.

Important Note

In both versions, the extended leg on the opposite side should not lift off the floor. Fig. 153 shows this error, which is caused by a lack of stretching ability.

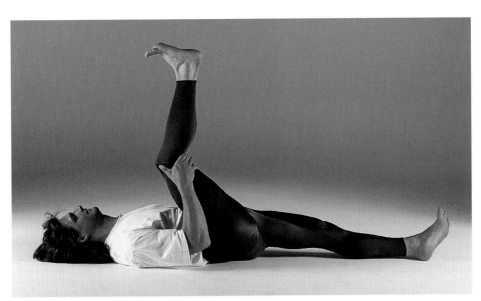

Fig. 152
Pull the tips of the toes of the foot pointing upward strongly toward the shin.

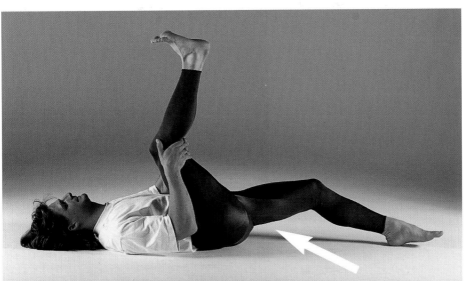

Fig. 153
How not to do it: The extended leg resting on the floor is bent.

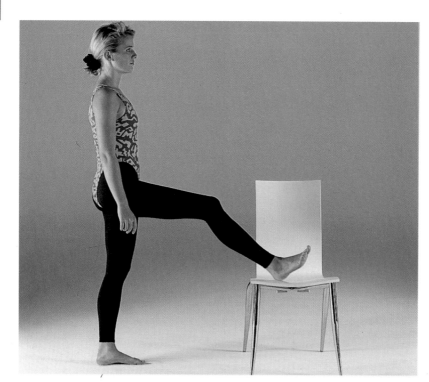

Fig. 154
Standing upright,
place the heel of
one foot on a
chair. Bend the leg
slightly at the
knee.

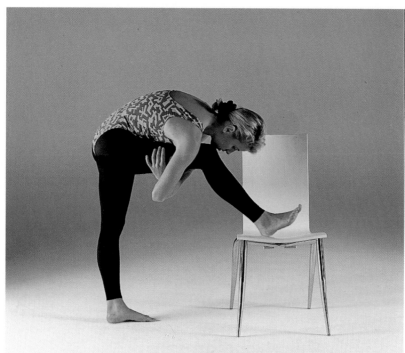

Fig. 155
Lower the torso to
rest on the thigh of
the raised leg. Pass
both hands around
the thigh.

Intensified Stretching

With the aid of a chair or a similar support, you can achieve a more intensive stretching in the back of the thighs.

Standing upright, place the heel of one foot on the chair. Bend the knee of that leg slightly. Pass both hands around the thigh in such a way that you can rest your torso on the leg. From this position, slowly shift the weight onto the supporting leg, while straightening the leg on the chair.

You need not straighten the knee fully, because the amount of movement is determined by the intensity of the stretch. (The straightened leg is not shown in the photo.)

Important Note

Fig. 157 shows another incorrect exercise that is frequently used. Here, there is no functional stretching of the back of the thighs, and it is the lumbar spine that is stressed.

You can also achieve the stretching in the previous exercise from a standing position without using a chair. In this case, you have to lower the torso further.

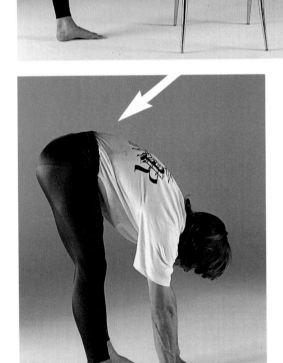

Fig. 156
Shift the weight onto the supporting leg, and straighten the bent knee as much as you can without causing a compensatory movement of the torso.

Fig. 157
How not to do it: **If you lack mobility, bending down to touch the floor with the legs straight puts a considerable strain on the lumbar spine.**

Variation

You can vary the exercise by turning your toes further inward or outward in the starting position. Perform the exercise as before, taking care that your torso doesn't lift off your thigh.

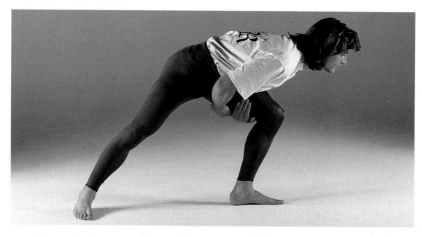

Fig. 158
Stand sideways with legs apart, placing one foot at a right angle to the other. Rest the torso on the thigh of the front leg, which is bent at the knee.

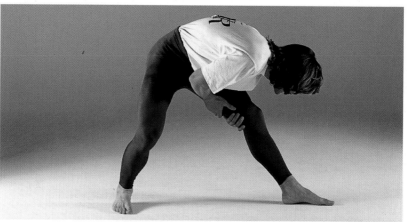

Fig. 159
Straighten the bent knee only as far as you can without causing a compensatory movement of the torso. The weight is shifted onto the leg with the bent knee in the process.

Fig. 160
A variation of the exercise: Point the toes of the leg that is to be turned further inward . . .

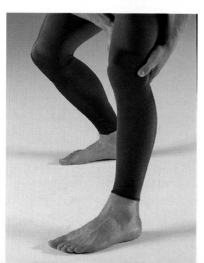

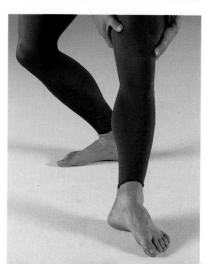

Fig. 161
. . .then further outward.

Stretching the Front of the Thighs and the Hip Flexors

Only some of the hip flexors can be tested without special aids. However, because this particular group of muscles suffers frequently from shortening, you should at least do one simple exercise. It has already been described in part at the beginning of the practical section (see page 14).

Testing the Stretching Ability of the Hip Flexors

Test
Lie on your back, and pull one leg as close to your rib cage as you can, while keeping your other leg extended on the floor. If you can flex the hip of the bent leg to its maximum without the other side of the body lifting off the floor, then its stretching ability is sufficient (Fig. 162). When the stretching ability is reduced, the straight leg is levered off the floor.

Exercise
Lie on your stomach, and grasp with one hand the instep of the foot on the same side, while keeping your other leg extended on the floor. The two bony protrusions of your pelvis are pressed hard against the floor. Then pull the heel toward the buttock with your hand, without abandoning the stabilization of the pelvis.

If you have difficulty stretching the front of the thighs this way, you should select one of the following exercises.

Important Note
Fig.164 shows a common incorrect exercise, which does not lead to stretching the front of the thighs specifically. The lumbar spine can again be subjected to heavy strain when doing this exercise.

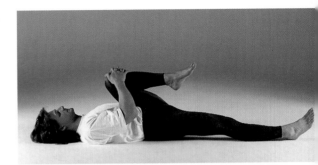

Fig. 162
Testing the stretching ability of the hip flexors: **Lie on your back, and grasp one knee with both hands, pulling the thigh as close to your torso as possible. Keep your other leg fully extended.**

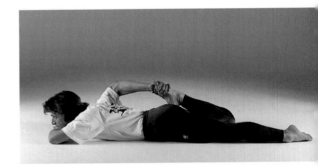

Fig. 163
Lie on your stomach, and grasp with one hand the instep of the foot on the same side. With the abdominal muscles tensed, pull the heel toward the buttock.

Fig. 164

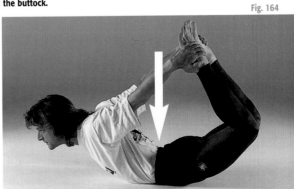

Variation

You can also stretch the muscles in the front of the thighs and the hip flexors effectively from a sitting position on a chair.

For this, you sit with one leg pulled up alongside the seat. You then perform the exercise as before, with one hand grasping the instep of the foot on the same side. Keep your other leg with its foot planted firmly on the floor.

Tense the abdominal muscles by pulling in the stomach. Only then pull the heel toward the buttock.

Important Note

Fig. 167 shows a compensatory movement that occurs if the abdominal muscles are not tensed enough. In this hollow-back position, no satisfactory stretching is possible.

Fig. 165

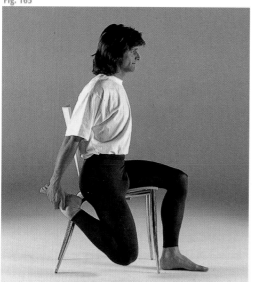

Fig 166

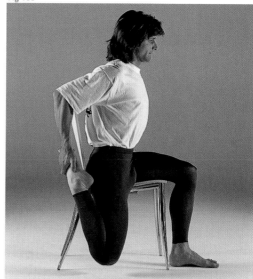

Fig. 165
Sit on a chair, and grasp with one hand the instep of the foot on the same side. Keep the sole of the other foot planted on the floor.

Fig. 166
With the abdominal muscles tensed, pull the heel toward the buttock.

Fig. 167
How not to do it: **The pelvis is not stabilized, and the lumbar spine slips out of position.**

Fig 167

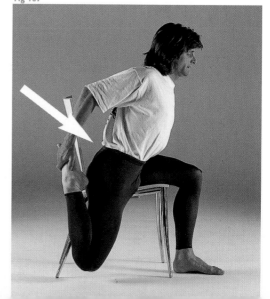

Exercise

With the following two exercises, you can achieve stretching positions first for some of the hip flexors and then for the muscles in the front of the thighs. Kneel on one knee, and place the front foot on the floor in such a way that you achieve a stable starting position.

Slowly shift the weight onto the front leg, and lower the hip of the back leg toward the floor.

Let your trunk go with the movement, but keep your spine as straight as possible.

You cannot always feel the stretching in the hip flexor distinctly, but don't abandon the exercise for this reason.

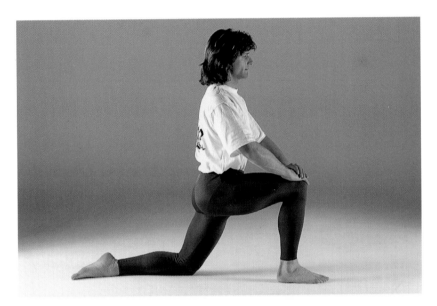

Fig. 168
Kneel on one knee, placing the sole of the front foot on the floor.

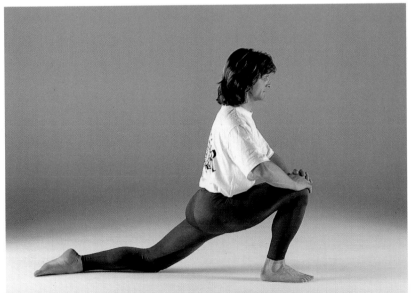

Fig. 169
Shift your weight onto the front leg, and straighten the hip joint of the back leg. Keep your spine straight.

Exercise

For the second stretching exercise, a certain amount of basic mobility is a prerequisite.

If you cannot achieve the position shown, then try one of the other stretching exercises for the front of the thigh instead. The stretching is achieved as before by shifting your weight forward, keeping your spine as straight as possible. Grip the instep of one foot with the hand on the same side, pulling the heel toward the buttock.

Fig.170

Grip the instep of one foot with the hand on that side. As you shift your weight, the heel is pulled toward the buttock.

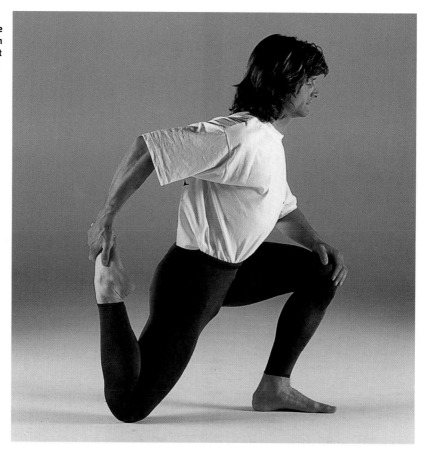

Exercise

Standing upright is the most precarious starting position you can take. It should only be chosen if the exercise in question can be done safely and with the necessary stability.

Grip one foot with the hand on the same side. Tense your abdominal muscles and stabilize the pelvis, so that you feel your stomach is being pulled in. The pull on the foot straightens your thigh in the hip joint and bends your knee very tightly.

During this exercise, don't let the torso bend forward or allow the lumbar spine to slip into a hollow-back position.

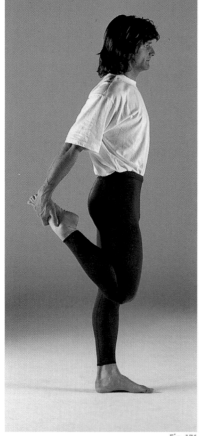

Fig. 171

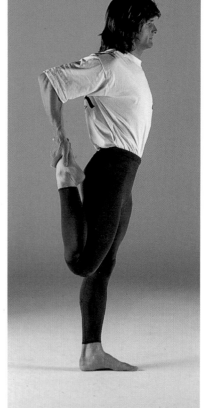

Fig. 171
Stand upright, and grip the instep of one foot with the hand on the same side.

Fig. 172
With tensed abdominal muscles, pull the heel toward the buttock.

Fig. 172   Fig. 173

Important Note

Fig. 173 shows a commonly used stretching exercise for the hip flexors and the muscles in the front of the thighs.

As with all stretching positions for this group of muscles, care should be taken that no compensatory movement of the lumbar spine occurs.

If, as shown in Fig. 173, the spine is shifted in this way, the exercise results in extra strain, and so should be avoided.

The stretching exercises for the hip flexors described here are useful supplements to any routine for the abdominal muscles.

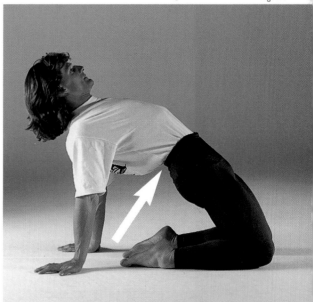

Fig. 174
Testing the stretching ability of the abductors of the thighs: **Lie on your back, and bend both legs to such an extent that the heels are as close to the buttocks as possible. Let the knees drop sideways.**

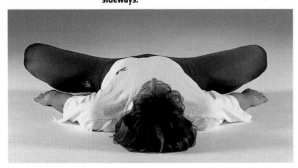

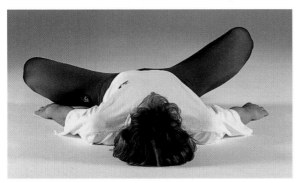

Fig. 175
Lack of stretching ability on one side: **If one knee doesn't drop as far as the other, then that side has reduced stretching ability.**

Fig. 176
Sit on the floor, and pull both heels toward the groin with your hands.

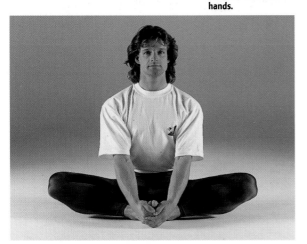

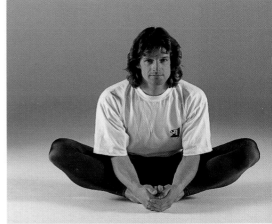

Stretching the Inside of the Thighs

The simplest way of testing the muscles in the inside of the thighs is to make a comparison between your left and right legs. You can get a good indication of a lack of stretch in the muscles from the intensity of the stretching feeling in the test position.

Testing the Stretching Ability of the Thigh Abductors

Test
Lie on your back, and bend both legs to such an extent that the heels are as close to the buttocks as possible. Let the knees drop sideways, and relax the muscles as much as you can. The further your knees drop, the better your stretching ability.

Fig. 174 shows a good final position. However, if one knee doesn't drop as far as the other (Fig. 175), and a stronger stretch can be felt on that side, then that side should be stretched more.

Fig. 177
Straighten the thoracic spine and lower the knees sideways toward the floor.

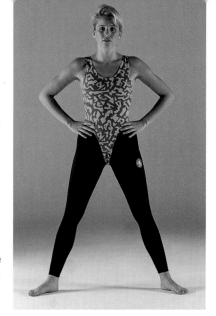

Fig. 178
Stand upright with your feet wide apart, and your toes turned slightly outward. Rest your hands on your hips.

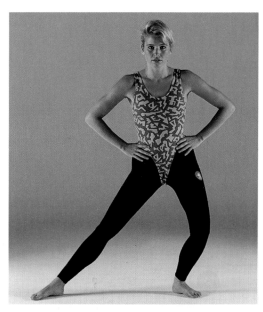

Fig. 179
Shift your weight onto one leg, while keeping the other leg straight. Your pelvis must remain in the erect position.

Exercise

Sit with your legs bent, and pull both feet toward the groin with your hands. Straighten the thoracic spine, which will give you the feeling of growing taller. Then lower your knees toward the floor, without abandoning the upright sitting position. This exercise only stretches certain sections of the specified muscle group, so you should always do the next exercise, as well.

Exercise

Stand upright with your legs apart in a straddle position, and your toes turned slightly outward. Shift your weight to one side, while keeping the leg on the opposite side extended.

Position the bent knee above the instep of the foot, and don't push it inward or outward. Keep your pelvis erect (this can easily be controlled by placing your hands on your hips). If you don't feel any stretching in the inside of the thigh, then move the legs further apart.

Important Note

Fig. 180 below shows a position that is often used. However, it doesn't produce the intended stretching.

Fig. 180
How not to do it: **The torso is lowered to rest on the bent leg, so the pelvis slips out of position.**

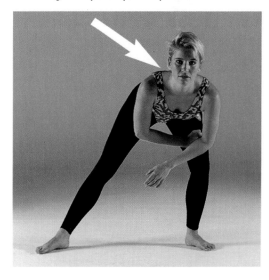

Intensified Stretching

You can achieve very intensive stretching of the thigh abductors with the following exercise: Support yourself on your forearms and your calves, with the pelvis so positioned that your hips are slightly more forward than your knees. Push your knees apart until you can feel a slight stretching in the inside of the thighs. The spine adopts a hollow-back position, which does not place any strain on the locomotor system in this starting position. By carefully shifting your weight backward, you initiate the stretching. Do not round your back.

Fig. 181
Support yourself on your calves and your forearms, with the hips slightly forward of the knees. Push your knees far enough apart to cause a slight stretching on the inside of the thighs.

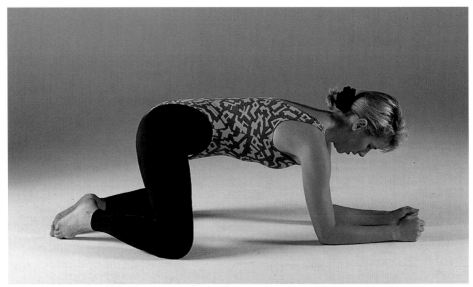

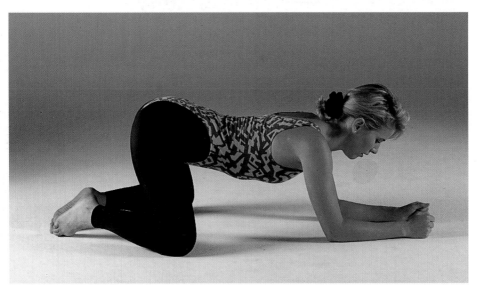

Fig. 182
The lumbar spine adopts a hollow position.

Rotating the Spine— Stretching the Muscles of the Buttocks and the Back

Exercise

Sit on the floor, and place one foot beside the knee of the extended leg. Rest the elbow of the arm on the opposite side on the outside of the bent knee. By pressing hard with your elbow against the bent leg, the thigh is pushed in the direction of your torso. The buttocks must not lift off the floor in the process.

Now turn the whole trunk in the opposite direction to the stretch, following this movement with your head. To secure better balance, place the free hand as support on the floor behind the buttocks.

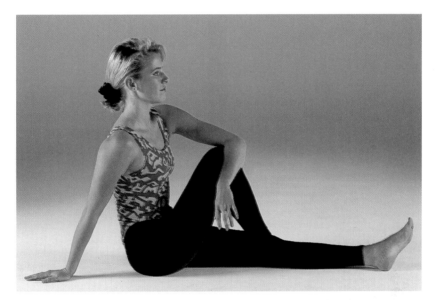

Fig. 183
In a sitting position, place one foot beside the knee of the extended leg. Rest the elbow on the same side as the extended leg on the outside of the bent knee. Support the torso with your free hand.

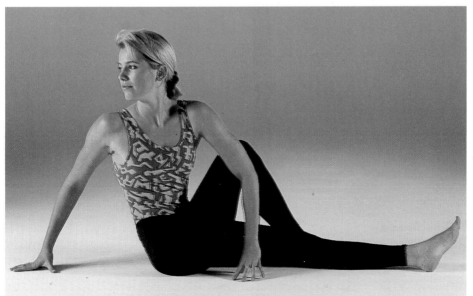

Fig. 184
Push the bent knee toward the torso by pressing with your elbow. Turn the trunk in a contrary motion, and follow it with your head.

Rounding the Spine— Stretching the Back Muscles

Exercise

Lie on your back, and bend both legs so that your thighs touch your torso. Grip the knees from the outside with both hands, pulling them apart further than the width of your hips. By pulling strongly on both legs, flex the hip joints more, and then lift your head and push it between the knees.

In the final position, your body should be curled up as tightly as possible. This position can also be used as a compensatory exercise after any of the toning exercises for the back muscles.

Fig. 185
Lie on your back, grip your knees with both hands, and draw your thighs close to your torso.

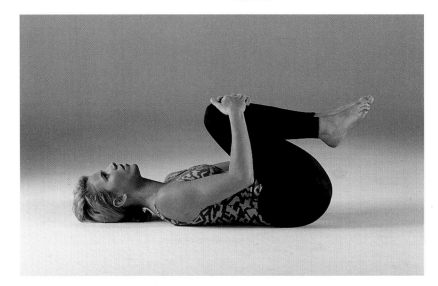

Fig. 186
Part your knees wide enough for your head to fit between them. Curl up your whole body as tightly as possible.

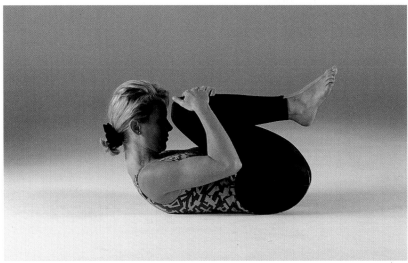

Rotating the Spine— Stretching the Back Muscles

Exercise

Lie on one side, and bend both legs at right angles, while keeping your torso straight. From this position, slowly move the top shoulder back. The top arm may remain bent, but you can also straighten it, as long as you don't find the stretching uncomfortable.

Keep your legs in the starting position, so that the bent knees don't lift off the floor. If you can do this exercise without effort, it can be made a little more difficult by varying it slightly, as will be described below.

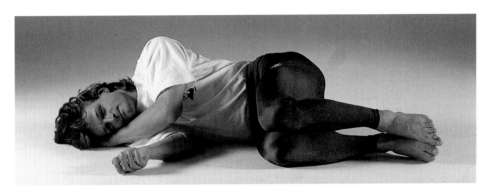

Fig. 187
Lie on one side, and bend both legs at right angles, while keeping the torso straight.

Fig. 188
Move the top shoulder slowly back, keeping your knees in the starting position.

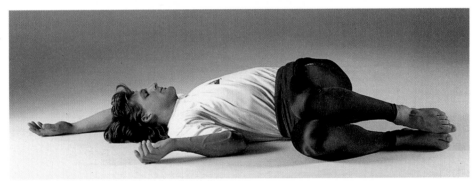

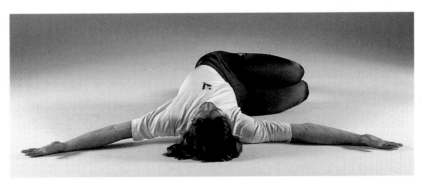

Fig. 189
A variation of the exercise: Straighten the top arm, and rest it beyond your head.

Intensified Stretch

Lie on one side, and bend your top leg, resting it on the other leg. Hold the knee on the floor with the hand of the bottom arm. Move the upper shoulder or extended arm backward as before. With the aid of a roll of foam material or a rolled-up mat, another stretching position is possible. Lie on one side, with the roll or mat placed under the thoracic spine. Bend the bottom leg in order to achieve a more stable starting position. Then lower your upper arm over your head toward the floor until the stretching can be felt in the top side of your body.

It's a good idea to hold these stretching positions for some time. The stretching can also be supported by breathing in such a way that the stretched side expands.

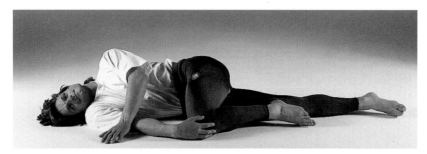

Fig. 190
Lie on one side with the bottom leg extended and the top one bent. Hold the bent knee on the floor with the hand of the bottom arm.

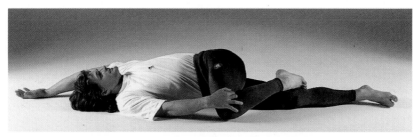

Fig. 191
Slowly move the upper shoulder backward, keeping the knee in the starting position.

Fig. 192
Lie on one side, with the spine supported by a roll just below the shoulder blades. Keep your body straight, and bend the bottom leg.

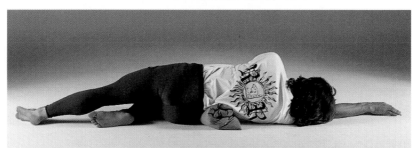

Fig. 193
Bring the upper arm over your head toward the floor as an extension of your body.

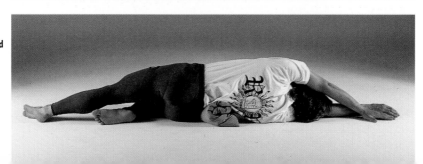

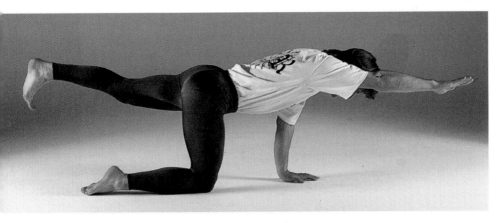

Fig. 194
Starting with your body supported on the calves and the hands, raise one leg and the arm on the opposite side into a horizontal position.

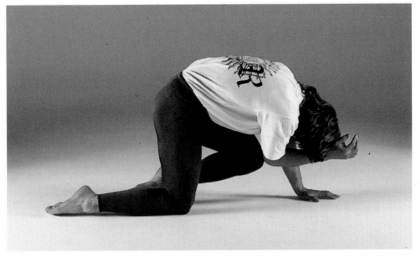

Fig. 195
Bring one elbow and the opposite knee together under the body, while rounding the spine.

Stabilizing and Mobilizing the Entire Spine

Exercise

A combined stabilizing and mobilizing exercise starts with the body supported on the calves and the palms of the hands or the fists (see page 50).

From this starting position, raise one leg and the diagonally opposite arm, so as to form an imaginary extension of the spine.

Be careful not to raise them above the horizontal, because this leads in most cases to undesirable compensatory movements of the spine. In the contrary movement, bring the elbow and the knee together under your body. You should round your back and keep the position steady.

This exercise can conveniently be combined with inhaling and exhaling, by breathing out in the rounded position and breathing in in the extended one.

Stretching the Muscles of the Chest and the Shoulder Girdle

Exercise

For the following stretching exercise, the previous support position on the calves and the hands must be altered. Slide your hands a long way forward over the floor, and let them come to rest a shoulders' width apart.

Push both shoulders down toward the floor, keeping your spine as straight as possible. The eyes remain fixed on the ground in this basic form.

You can vary the exercise by placing your hands wide apart on the floor and pushing only one shoulder at a time down toward the floor. Follow this movement with your eyes.

Fig. 196
From the kneeling position, lay your extended arms in front of your head as an extension of the spine. Push both shoulders down toward the floor.

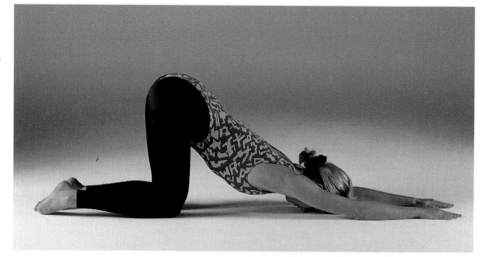

Fig. 197
Extend one arm and place it to one side, pushing the shoulder on that side down toward the floor. Support the torso with the other hand.

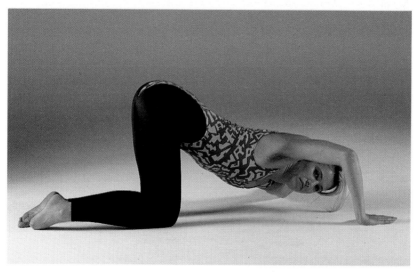

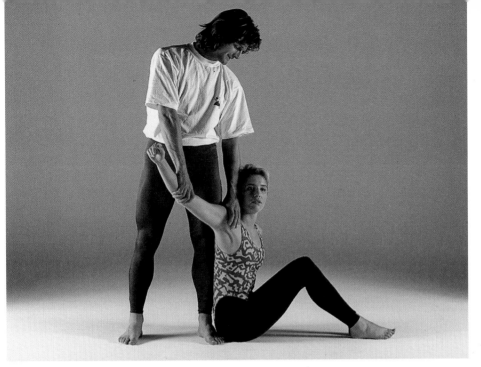

Fig. 198
Sit with your legs bent, while one arm is moved gently backward by your partner. Your partner's calf supports your spine, and one of his/her hands supports the shoulder on the same side.

Fig. 199
Both arms are pulled back by your partner at the same time.

Variations with the Help of a Partner

When stabilizing ability is poor, the last two exercises can easily lead to compensating movements of the spine. Hence, an alternative involving a partner is offered here.

Your spine is supported by one of your partner's legs, and your shoulder is held in position by one of his/her hands. The arm you have extended upward is drawn slowly back, and your partner stops the stretching when the thoracic spine begins to slip forward.

If the stretch can be performed in a controlled fashion—that is, without any change in the position of your spine—then it can also be done with both arms at the same time.

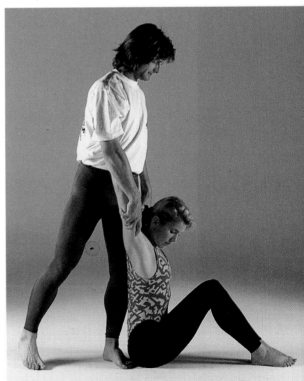

Stretching the Lateral Muscles of the Cervical Spine

The following stretching positions exercise the muscles of the cervical spine. They should all be done very slowly and without any effort. It is advisable to follow the stretching with a slight tensing of the muscles. You can do this easily by returning your head from the stretch position to the starting position against the resistance of the hand that is holding it.

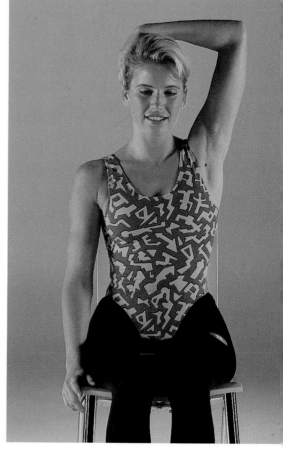

This resistance should lead to a slight tensing of the previously stretched muscles.

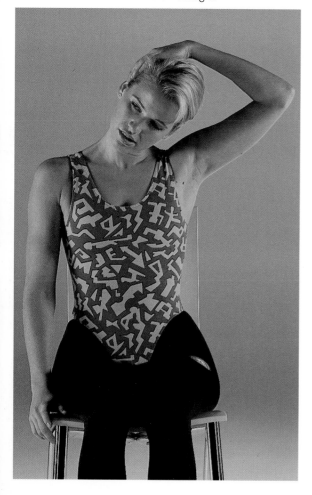

Fig. 200

Sit on a chair, and hold on to the seat with one hand, while reaching over your head to the opposite ear with the other hand.

Fig. 201

Pull your head slowly sideways with your hand.

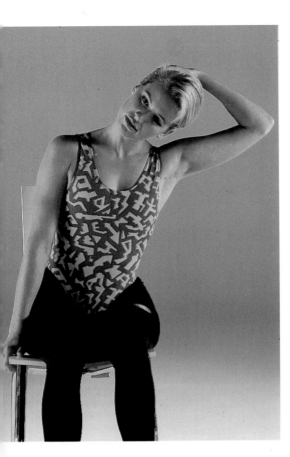

Fig. 202
Push your torso sideways on the chair with your supporting arm.

Fig. 203
A variation of the exercise: Reach behind your body to hold the opposite side of the chair back.

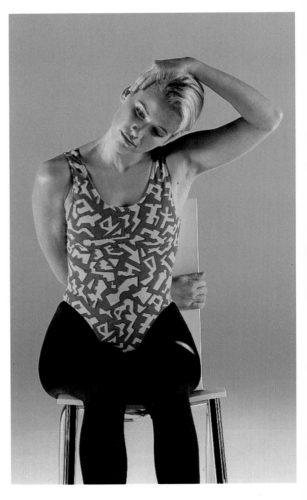

Exercise

Sit on a chair, and reach with one hand over your head to the ear on the opposite side. Hold on to the seat of the chair with your other hand. Pull your head gently sideways until you feel a slight stretching of the neck muscles. You can achieve further stretching by tilting your torso sideways, away from the hand holding on to the seat.

The intensity of the stretch depends on how much you tilt your body, and not on the pull on your head.

Variation

You can vary the exercise by reaching across behind your back with the supporting hand to grip the back of the chair.

Stretching the Neck Muscles

Exercise

You can also stretch your neck muscles while in a sitting position. Clasp your hands, and place them behind your head. Support your torso in an upright position against the back of the chair, while curving your cervical spine, vertebra by vertebra. When the gentle stretching begins, you can intensify it by applying a slight pressure with your hands on your head.

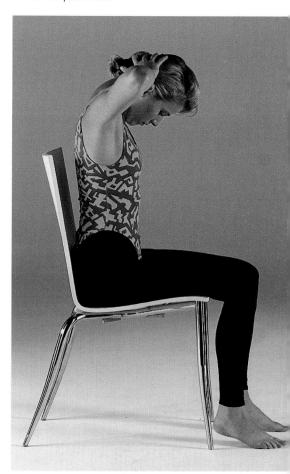

Fig. 204
Sit upright on a chair, and clasp your hands behind your head.

Fig. 205
Slowly curve your cervical spine, while applying pressure with your hands to intensify the stretch.

Variation

The same stretching exercise can be executed while sitting on the floor.

For this, your knees should be far enough apart for your elbows to fit between them. The stretching begins when you tilt your pelvis back out of its upright position.

Curve your cervical spine as before, and also round your thoracic spine.

The stretching spreads from your neck muscles to other parts of your spine.

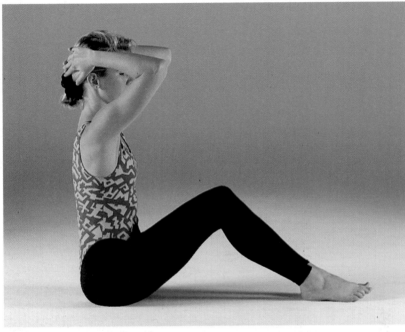

Fig. 206
Sit upright with your legs bent, and clasp your hands behind your head.

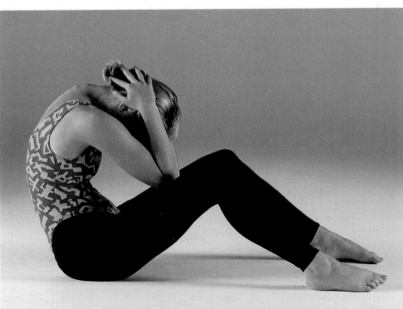

Fig. 207
Tilt your pelvis backward, round your back, and intensify the stretching with gentle pressure on your head.

Programs of Combined Exercise Routines

In the following 10 programs, the exercises described previously are grouped according to objective in order to form effective combinations. The method adopted here of combining stretching and toning exercises has proved to be a great success in practice.

It is recommended that you follow the instructions given to start with, and only later, when you are more familiar with these gentle exercises, vary them according to your particular needs.

The illustrations in the individual programs are intended only as reminders. If you think the particular version of an exercise given is too difficult or too easy, then you should follow the general principles for the exercises given on pages 12 to 13.

To make it easier to find the exercises in the main part of the book, the relevant page numbers are given each time in the pictorial chart.

To ensure correct procedure, it's important to follow the order depicted by the pictures. If, for instance, a stretching position is shown before a toning exercise and another one after, then this sequence should be followed.

Where an exercise is depicted in varying grades of difficulty, you should select from the column the version that you can do with confidence.

And where starting and final positions, and how not to do the exercise, are shown in one line, these are there as further reminders that you must set about the exercises the right way, because otherwise they will not be effective.

Program for Abdominal Muscles

Muscular System	Exercise Routine		
Exercise Content	Easy	Intermediate	Advanced
Abdominal muscles I	p. 19	p. 19	p. 24
Hip-flexors, stretching I		p. 74	
Abdominal muscles II	p. 19	p. 19	p. 24
Hip-flexors, stretching II		p. 76	
Pelvic stabilization I	p. 46	p. 55	p. 48
Back of thighs, stretching		p. 72	
Pelvic stabilization II	p. 44	p. 44	p. 45
Mobilization		p. 85	
Abdominal muscles III	p. 22	p. 22	p. 22
Back muscles, stretching		p. 82	

Easy Program for Beginners

Muscles Stressed	Toning	Strengthening	Toning
	Stretching Before Exercise		**Stretching After Exercise**
Abdominal muscles	p. 82	p. 17	p. 84
Stabilizing the pelvis	p. 73	p. 46	p. 73
Stabilizing the pelvis/shoulder girdle	p. 75	p. 53	p. 81
Abdominal muscles	p. 85	p. 19	p. 73
Stabilizing the shoulder girdle/hip joint	p. 79	p. 55	p. 86
Stabilizing the back muscles/hip joint	p. 73	p. 85	p. 70
Stabilizing the pelvis/shoulder girdle	p. 78	p. 44	p. 84
Back muscles	p. 81	p. 36	p. 82
Stabilizing the pelvis/leg muscles	p. 75	p. 47	p. 72
Back muscles	p. 86	p. 30	p. 31

Exercises Compensating for Sports That Overuse Certain Muscles

Muscular System / Exercise Content	Exercise Routine		
	Easy	**Intermediate**	**Advanced**
Straight abdominal muscles (toning)	p. 17	p. 15	p. 22
Back muscles (stretching)		p. 82	
Back muscles (toning)	p. 31	p. 85	p. 36
Hip-flexing muscles (stretching)		p. 75	
Buttock muscles (toning)	p. 46	p. 57	p. 62
Mobilization (general)		p. 85	
Stabilization (general)	p. 53	p. 54	p. 53
Muscles of the shoulder girdle (toning)	p. 47	p. 55	p. 56
Neck muscles (stretching)		p. 88	
Muscles of the torso (stabilizing)	p. 44	p. 44	p. 45

Supplementary Program for Endurance Training

Muscular System Exercise Content	Toning Exercise	Stretching Exercise	Wrong Version
Stabilizing the pelvis I	p. 56	p. 72	p. 71
Shoulder girdle I	p. 53	p. 74	p. 74
Stabilizing the torso I	p. 85	p. 85	
Stabilizing the pelvis II	p. 46	p. 73	p. 14
Shoulder girdle II	p. 53	p. 73	p. 73
Stabilizing the torso II	p. 30	p. 31	
Stabilizing the pelvis III	p. 47	p. 70	p. 71
Shoulder girdle III	p. 54	p. 76	p. 77
Stabilizing the torso III	p. 36	p. 84	
Stabilizing the torso IV	p. 62	p. 86	

Supplementary Program for Power Training

Muscular System Exercise Content	Starting Position	Final Position	Wrong Version
Back muscles I	p. 31	p. 31	
Abdominal muscles	p. 19	p. 19	
Back muscles II	p. 83	p. 84	
Hip flexors	p. 76	p. 76	p. 77
Muscles of the inner thighs	p. 72	p. 72	p. 71
Mobilization I	p. 85	p. 85	
Mobilization II	p. 82	p. 82	
Shoulder and neck muscles I	p. 88	p. 88	
Shoulder and neck muscles II	p.86	p.86	
Stabilization	p. 54	p. 54	p. 54

General Mobility Program

Muscular System / Exercise Content (Stretching)	Tensing Before Stretching	Stretching Exercise		Tensing After Stretching
Calves	p. 47	p. 66	p. 67	p. 53
Back of thighs	p. 47		p. 70	p. 54
Front of thighs	p. 53		p. 73	p. 46
Inside of thighs	p. 45		p. 79	p. 44
Hip flexors	p. 53		p. 75	p. 62
Back	p. 36		p. 83	p. 17
Shoulders	p. 54		p. 86	**p. 17**
Neck	p. 31		p. 88	p. 47
Shoulders/chest	p. 53		p. 86	p. 22
Back	p. 44		p. 82	p. 36

Spinal Program

Muscular System	Version of Exercise		Stretching
Exercise Content	**Easy**	**Advanced**	
Abdominal muscles	p. 19	p. 19	p. 74
Buttock muscles	p. 47	p. 57	p. 73
Back muscles	p. 85	**p. 37**	p. 81
Stabilizing the pelvis/shoulder girdle	p. 55	p. 57	p. 72
Abdominal muscles	p. 22	p. 24	p. 73
Buttock muscles	p. 44	p. 45	p. 81
Back muscles	p. 31	p. 36	p. 82
Stabilizing the shoulder girdle/pelvis	p. 54	p. 53	p. 75
Mobilization	p. 85	p. 85	p. 84
Stabilization	p. 56	p. 56	p. 66

General Toning Program

Muscular System	Version of Exercise		
Exercise Content	Easy	Intermediate	Advanced
Abdominal muscles	p. 19	p. 19	p. 24
Back muscles	p. 47	p. 85	p. 36
Stabilizing the shoulder girdle	p. 47	p. 55	p. 57
Buttock muscles	p. 47	p. 47	p. 62
Stabilizing the pelvis	p. 43	p. 44	p. 45
Abdominal muscles	p. 22	p. 22	p. 22
Back muscles	p. 31	p. 85	p. 37
Stabilizing the shoulder girdle	p. 53	p. 53	p. 54
Buttock muscles	p. 55	p. 55	p. 57
Stabilizing the pelvis	p. 56	p. 56	p. 47

Program for Backache

Muscular System / Exercise Content	Toning (T)	Stretching (S)	Wrong Version
T: Abdominal muscles / S: Back muscles	p. 19	p. 82	pp. 8, 71
T: Buttock muscles / S: Hip flexors	p. 47	p. 73	pp. 73, 77
T: Buttock muscles / S: Outside of thighs	p. 44	p. 81	p. 41
Mobilization	p. 85	p. 85	pp. 33, 71
T: Back muscles / S: Hip flexors	p. 36	p. 73	pp. 33, 73
T: Abdominal muscles / S: Back muscles	p. 19	p. 84	p. 8
T: Buttock muscles / S: Back of thighs	p. 62	p. 70	p. 71
Mobilization	p. 85	p. 85	pp. 33, 71
T: Back muscles / S: Hip flexors	p. 37	p. 74	pp. 73, 74
Stabilization	p. 54	p. 75	pp. 54, 74

Compensatory Program for Those Leading a Sedentary Life

Muscular System / Exercise Content	Starting Position	Final Position	Wrong Version
Calves I	p. 66	p. 66 · p. 67	p. 71
Back of thighs II	p. 70	p. 71	p. 71
Front of thighs	p. 74	p. 74	p. 74
Abdominal muscles	p. 19	p. 19	p. 8
Back muscles	p. 81	p. 81	p. 71
Buttock muscles	p. 46	p. 46	p. 33
Shoulder/neck muscles I	p. 88	p. 88	
Shoulder/chest muscles	p. 86	p. 86	
Shoulder/chest muscles II	p. 88	p. 89	
Stabilization	p. 31	p. 31	

Index